Study Guide to Accompany
Pharmacological Aspects of Nursing Care
Eighth Edition

Bonita E. Broyles, RN, BSN, EdD, PhD

Barry S. Reiss, BS, MS, PhD

Mary E. Evans RN, BSEd, MSN, FAAN, PhD

Prepared by
Valerie O'Toole Baker, RN, MSN, ACNS, BC
Prior edition written by Peggy S. Denning, RN, MSN, ADON

DELMAR
CENGAGE Learning·

Australia • Brazil • Japan • Korea • Mexico • Singapore • Spain • United Kingdom • United States

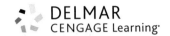
DELMAR
CENGAGE Learning·

Study Guide to accompany Pharmacological Aspects of Nursing Care, Eighth Edition
Bonita E. Broyles, Barry S. Reiss, Mary E. Evans
Prepared by: Valerie O'Toole Baker, RN, MSN, ACNS, BC

Vice President, Editorial: **Dave Garza**

Executive Editor: **Stephen Helba**

Senior Acquisitions Editor: **Maureen Rosener**

Managing Editor: **Marah Bellegarde**

Senior Product Manager: **Elisabeth F. Williams**

Editorial Assistant: **Samantha Miller**

Vice President, Career and Professional Marketing: **Jennifer Baker**

Senior Marketing Director: **Wendy Mapstone**

Executive Marketing Manager: **Michele McTighe**

Associate Marketing Manager: **Scott Chrysler**

Production Manager: **Andrew Crouth**

Content Project Manager: **Thomas Heffernan**

Senior Art Director: **Jack Pendleton**

Production Technology Analyst: **Patricia Allen**

For product information and technology assistance, contact us at
**Cengage Learning Customer & Sales Support,
1-800-354-9706**
For permission to use material from this text or product, submit all requests online at **www.cengage.com/permissions**.
Further permissions questions can be e-mailed to
permissionrequest@cengage.com

Library of Congress Control Number: 2011941348

ISBN-13: 978-1-4354-8918-9

ISBN-10: 1-4354-8918-7

Delmar
5 Maxwell Drive
Clifton Park, NY 12065-2919
USA

Cengage Learning is a leading provider of customized learning solutions with office locations around the globe, including Singapore, the United Kingdom, Australia, Mexico, Brazil, and Japan. Locate your local office at: **international.cengage.com/region**

Cengage Learning products are represented in Canada by Nelson Education, Ltd.

To learn more about Delmar, visit **www.cengage.com/delmar**

Purchase any of our products at your local college store or at our preferred online store **www.CengageBrain.com**

Printed in the United States of America
1 2 3 4 5 6 7 08 09 10 11

TABLE OF CONTENTS

PREFACE

The purpose of the *Study Guide to Accompany Pharmacological Aspects of Nursing Care,* Eighth Edition, is to help you learn, absorb, and retain difficult and often unfamiliar concepts in pharmacological nursing. This *Study Guide* will help reinforce major concepts as you review the central facts of each textbook chapter, and it will help you to develop the knowledge and skills you will need to succeed as a nurse in any health care setting.

Each chapter of the *Study Guide* has been thoroughly revised and reformatted to help you maximize your study time. Objectives are included so you understand at a glance the scope and coverage of the chapter. New Definition exercises test your knowledge and understanding of key terms in the chapter; you will be asked to write the definition to important phrases and terms. New Fill in the Blank questions require you to complete a sentence drawing on your knowledge of the content. Revised Multiple Choice questions quiz you on your grasp of material covered in the chapter. New Multiple Response questions follow the new NCLEX testing pattern in asking you to choose several correct answers from the choices listed. Updated Critical Thinking exercises take you one step further into problem solving and applying your skills to resolve real-life situations.

CHAPTER 1 Drugs/Agents and Factors Affecting Their Action

Objectives

After reading Chapter 1 of *Pharmacological Aspects of Nursing Care*, 8th edition, the student will be able to:

1. Describe the scope of the science of pharmacology.

2. Identify drug sources and provide an example of each.

3. Identify the properties of each of the following dosage forms: tablets, capsules, troches, suppositories, solutions, suspensions, emulsions, semisolid dosage forms (ointments, creams, and gels), transdermal patches, and parenterals (ampules, vials, and prefilled syringes).

4. Compare the significance of the chemical name, generic name, and brand name of a drug.

5. Discuss the meaning of each part of a "product insert" and a "patient package insert" (PPI).

6. Identify the component parts of a written prescription.

7. Identify the meaning of common abbreviations used in prescriptions.

8. Discuss the significance of each controlled substance schedule as defined in the Controlled Substances Act of 1970 (Title II of the Comprehensive Drug Abuse Prevention and Controlled Substances Act of 1970).

9. Describe Canadian drug legislation.

10. Briefly describe the review process employed by the FDA in evaluating the safety and effectiveness of nonprescription drug products.

11. Identify the significance of each of the four phases involved in the clinical testing of a new drug.

12. Describe the FDA Medical Products Reporting Program.

13. Describe the role of the nurse in the clinical testing of a new drug.

14. Describe the unique characteristics of each of the following drug information sources: *AHFS Drug Information*, *Physicians' Desk Reference*, *Drug Facts and Comparisons*, and *Handbook of Nonprescription Drugs*.

15. Discuss the significance of the following terms in the measurement of drug concentrations in the body: minimum effective concentration (MEC), minimum toxic concentration (MTC), plateau or steady-rate concentration, peak concentration, and trough concentration.

16. Discuss the significance of the term bioequivalent as it pertains to a drug product.

17. Compare the actions of agonist, partial agonist, and specific antagonist drugs.

18. Differentiate among each of the following adverse drug reactions: side effect, toxic effect, allergic reaction, idiosyncratic reaction, and teratogenic effect.

19. Describe the importance of each of the following factors in the passage of a drug through the body: stomach acidity, the solubility of drug in fat, drug-protein binding, microsomal enzymes, tubular secretion, and glomerular filtration.

20. Explain the relationship between the plasma concentration of a drug and its "drug half-life."

21. Describe the role of each of the following factors in determining a subject's pharmacological response to a drug: age, sex, body weight, body surface area, basal metabolic rate, disease states, genetic factors, placebo effect, time of administration, and tolerance.

22. Explain the significance of drug interactions, as well as physical and chemical incompatibilities of drugs in client care.

23. Discuss the history and significance of herbal medications.

24. Successfully complete the games and activities in the online student StudyWARE.

Definitions

Supply the definitions for the following terms.

1. pharmacokinetics _____

2. pharmacotherapeutics _____

3. pharmacogenetics _____

4. pharmacognosy _____

5. pharmacodynamics _____

Fill in the Blank

Write in the missing information.

1. _____ is the study of poisons and poisonings.

2. The most popular dosage form that is usually easiest to administer is the _____.

3. _____ are sweetened solutions that often are used to mask the unpleasant taste of certain drugs.

4. _____ are dispersions of fine droplets of an oil in water or water in oil.

5. If the administration of two or more drugs produces a pharmacological response that is greater than that which would be expected by the individual effects of each drug alone, the drugs are said to be acting _____.

Multiple Choice

Circle the best answer for each of the following questions. There is only one answer to each question.

1. The process by which a drug is carried from the absorption site to the site of action is known as
   A. drug distribution
   B. drug displacement
   C. drug half-life
   D. drug elimination

2. Paul and Walt are participants in a drug study. Both men are the same age and are similar in body height and weight. Both men are given a test dose of the experimental drug labeled "MED A." Walt develops an adverse reaction not seen in Paul or in any other study participant. Walt's reaction is an example of
   A. teratogenic effect
   B. idiosyncratic effect
   C. iatrogenic effect
   D. carcinogenic effect

3. The nurse identifies which of the following as the herb primarily used for the treatment of benign prostatic hypertrophy (BPH)?
   A. gingko
   B. echinacea
   C. ginseng
   D. saw palmetto

4. According to the Controlled Substance Act of 1970, controlled substances are classified into five different categories or schedules. Diazepam (Valium) falls into what category?
   A. Schedule II
   B. Schedule III
   C. Schedule IV
   D. Schedule V

5. Clinical studies performed on human subjects before marketing a product are divided into four phases. Which of the following is the phase involves broad clinical trials designed to evaluate drug usefulness in treating the disease for which it is claimed to be effective?
   A. Phase I
   B. Phase II
   C. Phase III
   D. Phase IV

6. Atorvastatin (Lipitor), a medication used to lower cholesterol, belongs to which group?
   A. curative drugs
   B. diagnostic drugs
   C. health maintenance drugs
   D. preventive drugs

7. Eddie, a college freshman, has been studying for midterms for the last week. To stay awake for the long group "cramming sessions," Eddie has been drinking all the coffee he can get his hands on. But Eddie has a mild case of asthma requiring an occasional puff of Ventolin, which he recently took. He is now experiencing shortness of breath and tachycardia. This is an example of

   A. drug interactions
   B. drug elimination
   C. drug metabolism
   D. drug absorption

8. By the time a drug becomes available to the public, it has been given several names. Which of the following identifies the structure of the drug?

   A. generic name
   B. chemical name
   C. brand name
   D. trade name

9. The nurse identifies which of the following herbs as most often used in the treatment of memory impairment?

   A. echinacea
   B. black cohash
   C. gingko
   D. valerian

10. The ability of this herbal to inhibit serotonin, dopamine, and norepinephrine reuptake in the central nervous system makes it popular for the treatment of mild to moderate depression.

   A. St. John's wort
   B. saw palmetto
   C. aloe
   D. garlic

Multiple Response

Circle the best answers for each of the following questions. More than one answer is correct.

1. Which of the following does the nurse identify as safe nursing practice for drug administration? Select all that apply.
   A. Administer enteric-coated products with milk.
   B. Crush enteric-coated tablets before administration.
   C. Shake suspensions immediately before use.
   D. Remove a previous transdermal patch before the next dosage patch is applied.
   E. Solutions administered in the eye must be sterile.
   F. Sublingual tablets should be placed in the inner lining of the cheek.

2. Which of the following statements about adverse drug effects does the nurse identify as true? Select all that apply.
   A. Adverse effects result from the normal pharmacologic effect of a drug.
   B. All drugs are capable of producing toxic effects.
   C. Allergic reactions are a result of the pharmacologic effects of the drug.
   D. Idiosyncratic reactions are the result of abnormal reactivity to a drug caused by genetic differences between the client and nonreacting individuals.
   E. A teratogenic drug is one that will cause a congenital defect in an infant whose mother took the drug while pregnant.
   F. Drug abuse develops when the client requires a higher dose or more frequent administration to produce the desired effect.

Critical Thinking Exercises

1. Discuss the procedures necessary for safe administration of any medication given via the transdermal method. Include proper dosage, patient preparation and precautions, nursing safety precautions, and proper disposal of the patch.

   _____

   _____

   _____

   _____

2. Name and describe each component of the health care providers' written prescription and the significance of each. Describe the difference between the written prescription and the hospital prescription.

_____

_____

_____

_____

3. Identify and describe the factors that contribute to the individual variations of drug responses.

_____

_____

_____

_____

4. Review the administration policies of controlled substances at the agency where you are having clinical experiences.

_____

_____

_____

_____

5. Review the nursing responsibilities when administering investigational drugs to clients.

_____

_____

_____

_____

6. Explore the use of herbal products in the treatment of clients with various conditions.

_____

_____

_____

_____

CHAPTER 2 *Principles and Methods of Drug Administration*

Objectives

After reading Chapter 2 of *Pharmacological Aspects of Nursing Care,* 8th edition, the student will be able to:

1. Relate the five steps of the nursing process to the administration of medications.
2. Discuss the "seven rights" of medication administration.
3. Discuss the importance of the right documentation.
4. Identify clients' rights regarding medication.
5. Define abbreviations commonly used in medication administration.
6. State the procedure for preparing drugs for parenteral administration from a multiple-dose vial.
7. Discuss The Joint Commission's, formerly the Joint Commission for Accreditation of Healthcare Organization (JCAHO), "Do Not Use" list with the Institute for Safe Medication Practices' (ISMP) "List of Error-Prone Abbreviations, Symbols, and Dose Designations" (The Joint Commission, 2009, Institute for Safe Medication Practice, 2007).
8. List the steps in withdrawing drugs from an ampule.
9. List three types of clients for whom the usual procedure of oral medication administration must be modified.
10. Describe the procedure for administration of medications by way of a nasogastric tube.
11. Select an appropriate injection site for administration of parenteral medications, being aware of developmental factors that could influence site selection.
12. Select an appropriate needle and syringe for various types of parenteral injections.
13. List sequentially the procedure to be used for intramuscular, subcutaneous, and intradermal injections.
14. List the steps for administering ear drops.
15. Discuss nursing actions related to the administration of medications for the treatment of gynecological health problems.
16. Apply the steps of the nursing process in client teaching.
17. Discuss a nursing process approach to fostering compliance with medication regimens.
18. Successfully complete the games and activities in the online student StudyWARE.

Definitions

Supply the definitions for the following terms.

1. intra-articular _____
2. intrathecal _____
3. medicated douches _____
4. intradermal _____
5. parenteral _____

Fill in the Blank

Write in the missing information.

1. The seven rights of medication administration are _____, _____, _____, _____, _____, _____, and _____.

2. When administering an oral antacid, the nurse will instruct the client to not eat or drink for _____.

3. The nurse will measure oral medications _____ to ensure accurate measurement.

4. The nurse administers subcutaneous insulin at a _____ degree angle.

5. When administering ear drops to an adult, the nurse will pull the pinna _____.

Multiple Choice

Circle the best answer for each of the following questions. There is only one answer to each question.

1. The nurse administers a medication via a nasogastric tube and most likely flushes the tube with how much fluid?
   A. 25–75 mL
   B. 10–20 mL
   C. 30–50 mL
   D. 5–30 mL

2. The first action the nurse should take before administration of an oral medication to a client is to
   A. check the client's identification bracelet
   B. wash his or her hands
   C. check the label on the medication three times
   D. open unit-dose packages

3. When administering the following types of oral medications, which should never be crushed before administration?
   A. capsules
   B. tablets
   C. chewables
   D. enteric coated

4. The nurse expects a client with anaphylaxis to exhibit which of the following?
   A. bradypnea
   B. hypothermia
   C. hypertension
   D. laryngeal edema

5. The preferred anatomical site for the injection of 1 mL or less of a clear, nonirritating solution is the
   A. dorsogluteal site
   B. deltoid site
   C. ventrogluteal site
   D. vastus lateralis site

6. It is most important for the nurse to rotate sites when clients are receiving frequent intramuscular injections because
   A. drug absorption is enhanced
   B. tissue integrity is adversely effected
   C. client preference is honored
   D. lipodystrophy is prevented

7. A client has just returned from the postanesthesia care unit and has an intravenous access device. The client is prescribed morphine sulfate via the intramuscular route for pain management. What action should the nurse take?
   A. Administer it as prescribed within the frequency parameters.
   B. Explain to the client that this is the prescribed route.
   C. Collaborate with the health care provider to change route of administration to IV.
   D. Suggest that a new nurse do the intramuscular injections "because it is good practice" for him or her.

8. A client is ordered an intramuscular injection of vitamin B$_{12}$. What should the nurse do to decrease the pain of this injection?
   A. Collaborate with the health care provider on a prescription for the local anesthetic-eutectic mixture of lidocaine and prilocaine (EMLA).
   B. Rub the area of the injection firmly with alcohol before administering.
   C. Administer the medication as quickly as possible.
   D. Administer the medication via the intravenous route.

9. The nurse is caring for a client who is receiving medications via a gastrostomy tube. The client is prescribed three medications to be administered at 10:00 AM. What action should the nurse take when administering these medications?
   A. Mix the medications together and flush the G-tube with normal saline after administering the medications.
   B. Crush medications, mix in sterile water, and then administer the medications together.
   C. Check the client's G-tube residual prior to administering the medications and discard the residual obtained.
   D. Administer each medication separately and flush the G-tube with water between each one.

10. The nurse is preparing to administer an intradermal turberculin skin test to a client. Which action should the nurse take during the administration?

    A. Insert the needle with the bevel pointed downward at a 10-degree angle.

    B. Insert the needle at a 15-degree angle with the bevel up.

    C. Insert the medication at a 45-degree angle, ensuring that the medication is absorbed.

    D. Be sure that you are using a 22-gauge, 1/2-inch needle.

Multiple Response

Circle the best answers for each of the following questions. More than one answer is correct.

1. When administering ear drops, the nurse will do which of the following? Select all that apply.

    A. Cool the medication to 95°F.

    B. Clean the inner ear with a cotton tip swab.

    C. Pull the pinna of the ear up and out for children under 3 years of age.

    D. Pull the pinna back and down for adults.

    E. Advise the client to remain in the same position for about 5 minutes following administration of the drug.

    F. When the client sits up, allow the remaining medication to flow out of the ear canal.

2. When administering an eye medication the nurse will do which of the following? Select all that apply.

    A. Place the medication on the cornea.

    B. Apply gloves before administering the medication.

    C. Place drops under the upper lid.

    D. Place drops into the center of the conjunctival sac.

    E. Perform hand hygiene.

    F. Wash hands after removing gloves.

Critical Thinking Exercises

1. Discuss the full impact of the "seven rights" of medication administration. Define these "seven rights" and the complications that can arise if any right is overlooked.

_____

_____

_____

_____

2. Describe the procedures for the administration of medications by injection, concentrating on intramuscular, intravenous, and subcutaneous. Name the injection sites, identify the anatomical landmarks, and identify when these particular sites are used.

_____

_____

_____

_____

3. Explore nursing interventions that may be used to enhance client compliance with medication therapy.

_____

_____

_____

_____

4. Practice various methods of medication administration by the parenteral and enteral route in the skills lab of your school.

_____

_____

_____

_____

CHAPTER 3 *Intravenous Drug Therapy*

Objectives

After reading Chapter 3 of *Pharmacological Aspects of Nursing Care*, 8th edition, the student will be able to:

1. Describe the nursing considerations in caring for a client receiving an intravenous infusion.

2. List in a stepwise manner the procedure for venipuncture.

3. Describe the procedure involved in administration of a drug intravenously by bolus injection through a primary intravenous setup.

4. Describe the administration of a drug intravenously by intravenous (IV) push through a maintenance port or a heparin lock.

5. Discuss the use of electronic infusion devices to monitor intravenous therapy.

6. Discuss the complications of intravenous therapy.

7. Apply the nursing process for clients receiving intravenous therapy.

8. Apply the appropriate nursing interventions for clients experiencing complications of intravenous therapy.

9. Calculate the rate of flow of intravenous infusions.

10. Successfully complete the games and activities in the online student StudyWARE.

Definitions

Supply the definitions for the following terms.

1. hydrostatic pressure _____

2. osmotic pressure _____

3. colloids _____

4. isotonic solutions _____

5. crystalloids _____

Fill in the Blank

Write in the missing information.

1. The nurse's highest priority during intravenous infusion therapy is _____.

2. _____ is the insertion of a needle into a vein.

3. _____ is the formation of a blood clot and inflammation of the vein.

4. When fluid being infused into a vein escapes from the vein to the surrounding tissue, it is called _____.

5. Complications of intravenous therapy include _____, which is the development of fever and chills associated with nausea, vomiting, and headache.

Multiple Choice

Circle the best answer for each of the following questions. There is only one answer to each question.

1. The nurse identifies this intravenous fluid as useful when the desired effect is to increase vascular volume and dehydrate the cells, causing them to shrink.

   A. isotonic
   B. hypertonic
   C. hypotonic
   D. hydrostatic

2. When administering medication via IV push (bolus), the nurse understands that the safest rate is

   A. 1 mL/min
   B. 0.5 mL/min
   C. 1.5 mL/min
   D. 2 mL/min

3. After administering a medication via IV push, the nurse understands that therapeutic or adverse effects will most likely be seen

   A. within 5 to 10 minutes
   B. within 30 minutes
   C. by the end of his or her shift
   D. immediately

4. The nurse identifies the intravenous solution that has the same osmolality as body fluids and does not alter plasma osmolality as

   A. hypertonic solution
   B. hypotonic solution
   C. isotonic solution
   D. hydrating solution

5. A client is ordered colloid solutions. Which of the following will the nurse question?

   A. albumin
   B. plasmanate
   C. Ringer's Lactate
   D. dextran

6. One of the most common electrolytes added to intravenous fluids is potassium. When the natural balance of this electrolyte is disrupted, cardiac disturbances occur that may prove fatal. Knowing this, the nurse takes special care to ensure that potassium remains within this range.

   A. 2.0–4.5 mEq/L
   B. 3.5–5.0 mEq/L
   C. 4.0–6.5 mEq/L
   D. 1.5–3.0 mEq/L

7. The nurse identifies which of the following solutions as an isotonic solution?

   A. D5 0.9 NaCl
   B. D5 Ringer's solution
   C. 0.45 NaCl
   D. Dextran 40 and D5W

8. Tissue damage, breakdown, and sloughing that occur following infiltration of an IV delivering a toxic medication is called

   A. infiltration
   B. necrosis
   C. extravasation
   D. thrombophlebitis

9. It is most important for the nurse monitoring a client receiving crystalloids to assess for the development of

   A. pulmonary edema
   B. dehydration
   C. renal failure
   D. allergic reaction

10. When administering lactated Ringer's solution to a client, it is most important for the nurse to assess the client for the development of

    A. hypernatremia
    B. hyperkalemia
    C. hypercalcemia
    D. hypermagnesemia

Multiple Response

Circle the best answers for each of the following questions. More than one answer is correct.

1. When working with a client who develops a pyrogenic reaction, the nurse should do which of the following? Select all that apply.

   A. Administer acetaminophen and continue the infusion.
   B. Administer an antiemetic agent and continue the infusion.
   C. Document the findings and continue to monitor the client.

D. Discontinue the infusion.
E. Send the fluid to the pharmacy.
F. Send the intravenous administration set to the pharmacy.

2. When infusing intravenous fluids and medications, the nurse will do which of the following? Select all that apply.
   A. Discard intralipids that are cloudy.
   B. Prime all administration setups before use.
   C. Check intravenous patency after administering any medication.
   D. Administer intravenous bolus medications at 1 mL/min.
   E. Document intake and output on an hourly basis.
   F. Use filters when administering total parenteral nutrition.

Critical Thinking Exercises

1. Discuss the procedure (step by step) for initiating intravenous therapy on a client, including the correct procedure for equipment setup.

2. Explain the procedure for using an electronic infusion device.

3. Explain the procedure for administering an IV push (bolus) medication and the possible complications that may occur with this medication delivery method.

4. Discuss client teaching needs for use of intravenous therapy in the home.

5. Discuss assessment, nursing diagnoses, plan of care, potential problems, interventions, and evaluation of intravenous therapy.

_____

_____

_____

_____

_____

6. Explore nursing interventions to prevent and treat complications associated with intravenous therapy.

_____

_____

_____

_____

_____

CHAPTER 4 *Calculating Medication Dosages*

Objectives

After reading Chapter 4 of *Pharmacological Aspects of Nursing Care*, 8th edition, the student will be able to:

1. Interpret a medication prescription accurately.
2. Convert quantities stated in household units to their equivalent units in the metric system.
3. Convert quantities stated in metric/SI International System units to other units within that system (e.g., grams, milligrams).
4. Set up valid proportions to perform calculations required in administering medications.
5. Calculate quantities to be administered when prescribed in fractional doses.
6. Calculate safe dosages for infants and children.
7. Calculate dosages for individual clients given the client's weight and/or height and the recommended dose.
8. Perform calculations necessary for the infusion of intravenous (IV) medications.
9. Discuss steps to decrease errors in interpreting the strength of drugs from the written prescription.
10. Successfully complete the games and activities in the online student StudyWARE.

Definitions

Supply the definitions for the following terms.

1. ratio _____

2. proportion _____

3. gram _____

4. liter _____

Fill in the Blank

Write in the missing information.

1. To convert a quantity in the metric system to a larger unit (e.g., milligrams to grams), move the decimal point to the _____.
2. To convert a quantity in the metric system to a smaller unit (e.g., grams to milligrams), move the decimal point to the _____.
3. The apothecary system is based upon _____.
4. Pediatric dosages are often calculated as _____ of body weight in a given period of time.
5. A _____ is a chart that uses the height and weight of the client to estimate his or her body surface area (BSA) in square meters (m^2).

Practice Problems

1. The health care provider prescribes penicillin 500,000 units IV every 6 hours. You have penicillin 1,000,000 units/mL on hand. How many mL will you give?

2. The health care provider prescribes nitroglycerin gr 1/150 sublingual every 5 minutes times three doses. The vial in the medication cart contains nitroglycerin 0.04 mg. How many tablets will you give per dose?

3. Theophylline 100 mg po every 8 hours is prescribed. You have theophylline 400 mg/5 mL available. How much would you give?

4. The client you are caring for has a seizure disorder and needs phenytoin (Dilantin) 0.2 g po tid. The pharmacy has sent phenytoin (Dilantin) 100 mg/4 mL. How much will you give for each dose?

5. The client has a wound that needs to be irrigated with 0.25 L of sterile saline. The saline is in a one-liter bottle. How many milliliters will you use?

6. The client is to receive penicillin 2 g po now. Penicillin 500 mg/capsule is available. How many capsules will you give?

7. The health care provider asks for Drug A 12.5 mg be given to his or her client every morning. The label says Drug A 25 mg/tablet. What is the correct dose?

8. A prescription reads: K-tabs 40 meq followed by 30 mL water. The label says K-tabs 20 meq/tab. What is the correct dose?

9. An IV prescription says "add aminophylline 0.3 g to existing IV fluids." The vial is labeled aminophylline 500 mg/20mL. How much will you add?

10. A 10-kg client needs to have 1 mg/kg of Drug B. How much does the client need over 24 hours? If the amount is to be divided into two equal doses, how much is a single dose?

11. Heparin 2500 units, administered subcutaneously, is prescribed. The vial is labeled heparin 5000 units/mL. How much will you administer?

12. A medication prescription calls for 1000 mL normal saline (NS) to be administered in 5 hours. The drop factor is 15. How many drops per minute will the saline be infused?

13. An infant is to receive 50 mL of 4% dextrose via water IV in 4 hours. At what hourly rate should the nurse set the IV infusion pump to administer this fluid?

14. 1000 mL D5W are to be given at a rate of 21 gtt/min with a drop factor of 10 gtt/mL. How long will the infusion last?

15. An IV infusion of 80 mg of gentamicin in 100 mL of D5W is to infuse in 30 minutes through the client's central venous access device. At what hourly rate would the nurse program the IV infusion pump to administer the gentamicin in 30 minutes?

Critical Thinking Exercises

1. Read the manufacturer's suggested dosage information found in the package insert for a selected medication. Determine if your client has been receiving a therapeutic dose.

_____

_____

_____

_____

2. What would be the first action you would take if you calculated a drug dose and found that the dose prescribed was too high for the patient?

_____

_____

_____

_____

3. What factors might the nurse need to be aware of before administering medication to a client?

_____

_____

_____

_____

4. Discuss how the following medication errors could occur and how to prevent them: administering the wrong dose, administering an extra dose, omitting the dose, administering an unordered drug, administering by the incorrect route, and administering at the incorrect time.

_____

_____

_____

_____

CHAPTER 5 Drug Therapy for Pediatric Clients

Objectives

After reading Chapter 5 of *Pharmacological Aspects of Nursing Care*, 8th edition, the student will be able to:

1. Discuss anatomical and physiological factors that may result in altered drug effects in children.
2. Describe how pediatric dosages may be calculated.
3. Discuss need for caregiver consent prior to any procedures performed on minors.
4. Apply the nursing process as related to the administration of medications to children.
5. Discuss general guidelines to use in teaching children about their drug therapy.
6. Apply the nursing process as related to the prevention of accidental poisoning in children.
7. Successfully complete the games and activities in the online student StudyWARE.

Definitions

Supply the definitions for the following terms.

1. syrup of ipecac _previously used to induce vomitting, in the treatment of vomitting_
2. activated charcoal or magnesium _agents used by healthcare to prevent gastric absorption of poisons_
3. juniper oil _herb - diuretic_

Fill in the Blank

Write in the missing information.

1. It is essential to use topical products _sparingly_ in infants and to monitor children for the development of both local and systemic adverse effects related to excessive absorption of the applied drug to the skin.
2. _Renal_ excretion is the primary pathway of elimination for most drugs.
3. _Electronic Infusion Devices_ are often used to ensure accurate administration of intravenous fluids to children.

Multiple Choice

Circle the best answer for each of the following questions. There is only one answer to each question.

1. The nurse identifies the process by which drugs are excreted through the renal system as
   - A. glomerular filtration
   - B. passive tubular secretion
   - C. active tubular reabsorption
   - D. biotransformation

2. Drugs are metabolized enzymes, which promote elimination of that drug. The enzymes are produced by
   - A. the spleen
   - B. the liver
   - C. the kidneys
   - D. the pancreas

3. What is considered a "normal" adult weight for drug calculation purposes?
   - A. 120 lbs.
   - B. 130 lbs.
   - C. 150 lbs.
   - D. 100 lbs.

4. The nurse is using a nomogram that contains both height and weight. The data correlate fairly well to appropriate pediatric dosages. The nurse identifies which of the following statements as being true?

   A. Using only weights provides adequate dosing information.
   B. Nomograms are generally accurate only after the maturation of liver and kidney function has been attained.
   C. Not all medications are able to cross the blood-brain barrier.
   D. Nomograms are accurate for all levels of pediatric clients.

5. The nurse identifies the preferred intramuscular injection site for infants as the

   A. gluteus maximus
   B. tibialis anterior
   C. deltoid
   D. vastus lateralis

6. The nurse identifies the preferred method of reducing accidental poisonings in children as ~~Wrong in back of book~~

   A. use of syrup of ipecac
   B. prophylactic use of activated charcoal
   C. prevention
   D. use of magnesium sulfate

7. When preparing to administer a medication to an infant or a child, it is most important for the nurse to consider the infant's or child's

   A. age
   B. medical history
   C. prior experience taking medications
   D. developmental level

8. When administering medications to infants and children, the nurse understands they are most at risk for complications related to the administration of medications due to

   A. their small size and immature renal system
   B. their immature neurological system
   C. family history of medication use
   D. their immature respiratory system

9. A parent's involvement when infants or children younger than age 2 are to receive medication should be based on

   A. the health care provider's request
   B. the principle that children should always be held by the parent for medication administration
   C. the convenience for the nurse
   D. the parent's comfort level with being actively involved

10. Which of the following statements about the use of herbals by parents for health maintenance of their children does the nurse identify as being true?

    A. The effects on children are the same as the effects on adults.
    B. Use of buckthorn in children may cause clinically significant dehydration.
    C. Because these products are natural, children are not allergic to them.
    D. Because these products are derived from plants, children cannot overdose on them.

Multiple Response

Choose the best answers for each of the following questions. More than one answer is correct.

1. When administering a rectal suppository to an infant, the nurse will do which of the following? Select all that apply.

   A. Wash hands.
   B. Obtain an oil-based lubricant.
   C. Position the child on his or her abdomen.
   D. Use the index finger to insert the suppository.
   E. Advance the suppository past the anal sphincter.
   F. Withdraw finger and press the buttocks together for a few minutes.

2. When administering medications to children, the nurse will do which of the following? Select all that apply.

   A. Establish a trusting relationship with the child.
   B. Use a firm but kind approach.
   C. Mix medications into essential foods.
   D. Mix medications into milk.
   E. Tell the child the medication is candy.
   F. Punish the child when he or she is uncooperative.

Critical Thinking Exercises

1. What factors are important to consider before administering drug therapy to children, and why are these important?

_____

_____

_____

_____

2. Discuss the major factors that govern medication administration in children.

_____

_____

_____

_____

3. Create a visual presentation of the differences between children and adults in administration, metabolism, muscle mass, and excretion of medications.

_____

_____

_____

_____

4. Discuss the safety factors involved in administering oral medications to infants.

_____

_____

_____

_____

CHAPTER 6 *Drug Therapy for Older Adult Clients*

Objectives

After reading Chapter 6 of *Pharmacological Aspects of Nursing Care*, 8th edition, the student will be able to:

1. Discuss anatomical and physiological factors that may result in altered drug effects in the older adult.
2. Discuss social and environmental factors related to drug problems in the older adult.
3. Describe the assessment of older persons who are using medications.
4. Apply the nursing process related to the administration of medications to older adult clients.
5. Discuss general guidelines to use in teaching the older adult about drug therapy.
6. Successfully complete the games and activities in the online student StudyWARE.

Definitions

Supply the definitions for the following terms.

1. biotransformation _____
2. creatinine clearance _____
3. congestive heart disease _____

Fill in the Blank

Write in the missing information.

1. With advancing age, there is a ___reduction___ in the amount of hydrochloric acid produced in the stomach.
2. With advancing age, there is generally a ___decline___ in the body's ability to transform active drugs into inactive metabolites.
3. With aging, there is a gradual reduction in ___renal function___ that may significantly affect the safe and effective use of drugs.

Multiple Choice

Circle the best answer for each of the following questions. There is only one answer to each question.

1. When working with older adults, the nurse realizes that the process that helps to transform active drugs into inactive _____ declines with age.

    A. enzymes
    B. metabolites
    C. purines
    D. biotransformation

2. In older adults, most drugs are eliminated by the

    A. kidney
    B. liver
    C. sigmoid colon
    D. skin

3. Which of the following statements about self-medication practices in older adults does the nurse identify as being true?

    A. Many older adults are frequent users of laxatives.
    B. Older adults never share medications with friends.
    C. Older adults are at a lower risk of drug reactions because they are closely monitored.
    D. Provision of reading materials to an older adult ensures understanding of the medication.

4. When working with older adults, the nurse realizes that the absorption of drugs

A. is increased due to increased bile production   C. is the same as in younger adults

B. is decreased due to decreased gastric acidity   D. is decreased due to greater production of hydrochloric acid

5. The nurse assesses older adults for cumulative effects of drugs because

A. of increased glomerular filtration rate   C. topical absorption is faster

B. of decreased levels of digestive enzymes   D. glomerular filtration decreases by 40–50%

6. When working with older adults, the nurse uses caution because total body water is reduced, resulting in

A. decreased distribution of water-soluble medications   C. decreased absorption of all medications

B. increased distribution of fat-soluble medications   D. decreased number of intact nephrons

7. The nurse identifies that as a client ages, the blood flow to the intestines and kidneys

A. increases   C. remains the same

B. decreases   D. equalizes

8. When teaching the older adult about treatment of Type 2 diabetes, it is most important for the nurse to first

A. demonstrate the procedure for intradermal medication administration

B. demonstrate how to withdraw medication from an ampule

C. assess the client for disabilities and sensory functioning

D. have client repeat back the demonstration for administering the medication

9. Which of the following does the nurse identify as a factor related to drug problems in older adults?

A. Medication problems decrease with the use of multiple drugs.

B. As the number of drugs taken increases, the number of medication errors decreases.

C. Drug hoarding is not a problem with older adult clients.

D. Loss of recent memory can affect self-care.

10. Drug absorption in the older adult client is affected by

A. increased production of hydrochloric acid in the stomach

B. fast gastric emptying rate

C. increased muscle tone of the lower intestinal tract

D. reduced blood flow to the intestinal tract

Multiple Response

Circle the best answers for each of the following questions. More than one answer is correct.

1. When administering drugs to the elderly, the nurse will do which of the following? Select all that apply.

A. Follow the seven rights.

B. Place the client in the supine position to administer oral medications.

C. Use liquid dosage forms if the client has difficulty with tablets.

D. Use the liquid dose forms if the client has difficulty with capsules.

E. Use the deltoid as the preferred site for intramuscular injections.

F. Monitor older adults receiving intravenous infusions for fluid overload.

2. When teaching the older adult about the use of medications, the nurse will do which of the following? Select all that apply.

A. Encourage the client to share medications with family members.

B. Teach someone close to the client about the drug therapy.

C. Relate learning to previous life experiences.

D. Keep the teaching sessions brief.

E. Inform the client that because of age he or she will not have an adverse reaction to the medication.

F. Tell the client to only take half of the prescribed medication because his or her body is not able to excrete the medication.

Critical Thinking Exercises

1. Discuss the procedures necessary for the safe administration of any medication given to older adults. Include proper dosage, client teaching, nursing safety precautions, and proper documentation.

   _____

   _____

   _____

   _____

2. Develop a protocol or method to help an older adult coordinate daily medications. Include any over-the-counter medications taken on a regular basis.

   _____

   _____

   _____

   _____

3. Identify and describe the factors that contribute to the individual variations of drug responses among older adults.

   _____

   _____

   _____

   _____

4. Discuss nursing interventions to encourage compliance by older adults with medication regimens.

   _____

   _____

   _____

   _____

CHAPTER 7 *Antibacterial Agents and Antiviral Agents*

Objectives

After reading Chapter 7 of *Pharmacological Aspects of Nursing Care,* 8th edition, the student will be able to:

1. Discuss factors determining the selection of an antimicrobial agent for the treatment of an infection.
2. Differentiate between a bactericidal and bacteriostatic antimicrobial agent and describe when the use of each would be appropriate.
3. Describe four ways in which antimicrobial agents in general may act in exerting therapeutic actions.
4. Differentiate between narrow- and broad-spectrum antimicrobial agents and explain when each would be appropriate to use.
5. Describe the major classes of antibacterial agents and the drugs found in each class.
6. Discuss the major adverse effects associated with the use of each class of antibacterial agents.
7. Discuss the drug interactions associated with antibacterial agents.
8. Compare the difference between the therapeutic actions of antibacterial agents and the action of antiviral agents.
9. Discuss the major adverse effects associated with the use of antiviral agents.
10. Discuss the drug interactions associated with antiviral agents.
11. Discuss the use of the nursing process in the administration of each class of antibacterial agent and in the administration of antiviral agents.
12. Discuss the use of the nursing process in the administration of antiviral agents.
13. Apply the steps necessary to prepare an antibiotic solution from a powder.
14. Successfully complete the games and activities in the online student StudyWARE.

Definitions

Supply the definitions for the following terms.

1. host _____
2. mode of transmission _____
3. reservoir _____
4. portal of exit _____
5. portal of entry _____
6. infectious agent _____
7. antibacterial agents _____
8. bacteriostatic agents _____
9. broad spectrum or extended spectrum _____
10. bacteriocidal agents _____
11. viruses _____
12. gram stain _____

Fill in the Blank

Write in the missing information.

1. The factors that may increase the susceptibility of the body to infection include _____, _____ _____, _____, _____, _____, and _____.

2. _____ agents have a killing action on the microbial agent, and _____ agents simply inhibit growth of bacteria.

3. _____ are among the simplest living organisms.

4. Hypersensitivity reactions may be manifested as _____, _____, _____, _____, _____.

5. The _____ are among the oldest antibiotics used.

6. The _____ group of antibiotics is chemically and pharmacologically related to the penicillins, were developed due the acquired bacterial resistance to penicillins, and are the antibacterial agents most commonly prescribed today.

7. The _____ have a tendency to produce toxicity involving bone and tooth enamel, photosensitivity, and the likelihood of superinfection with prolonged or repeated administration.

8. The _____ include erythromycin, and are primarily used for oral therapy of respiratory, gastrointestinal, urinary, skin, and soft tissue infections caused by gram-positive and some gram-negative organisms.

9. Fluroquinolones are broad-spectrum antibiotics that are effective against gram-negative microorganisms, especially _____.

10. During the past several decades, tuberculosis has again emerged as a serious disease, particularly among members of the population with _____.

11. Treatment for Lyme disease most often consists of oral administration of _____or_____.

12. Hansen's disease is also known as _____.

Multiple Choice

Circle the best answer for each of the following questions. There is only one answer to each question.

1. A client is traveling to a third world country as part of her job requirements. The nurse anticipates the administration of which of the following drugs as being prescribed for the client to take starting 1–2 days before her trip?
   A. erythromycin estolate
   B. doxycycline hyclate
   C. amikacin sulfate
   D. chloramphenicol

2. A new nurse is administering vancomycin intravenously. The supervising nurse needs to intervene if the new nurse
   A. administers the IV dose over 30 minutes
   B. obtains baseline renal function
   C. uses a central line for infusion of the medication
   D. assesses the client for ototoxicity

3. When administering aminoglycosides, it is most important for the nurse to monitor the client for which of the following adverse effects?
   A. vomiting
   B. hepatotoxicity
   C. diarrhea
   D. ototoxicity

4. The nurse associates the development of red man syndrome as most likely the result of administration of which of the following?

   A. sulfadiazine

   B. vancomycin

   C. rifampin

   D. acyclovir

5. Which of the following broad-spectrum agents does the nurse identify with the adverse effects of photosensitivity and possible damage to the tooth enamel?

   A. nosocomial infection

   B. synergistic infection

   C. superinfection

   D. iatragenic reaction

6. Which of the following broad-spectrum agents does the nurse identify with the adverse effects of photosensitivity and possible damage to the tooth enamel?

   A. metronadazole

   B. azithromycin

   C. norfloxacin

   D. tetracycline

7. A client has a tick bite from the spirochete *Borrelia burgdorferi*. The nurse identifies the most likely result of this tick bite is the possible development of

   A. rheumatoid arthritis

   B. tuberculosis

   C. Lyme disease

   D. Rocky Mountain spotted fever

8. A client has been diagnosed with active tuberculosis. The nurse anticipates drug therapy for the client to most likely include which of the following?

   A. ceftazidime and tetracycline

   B. isoniazid and rifampin

   C. penicillin and amoxicillin

   D. gentamycin and vancomycin

9. A client has herpes simplex-1 virus. The nurse identifies which of the following as the mostly effective drug for use with this client?

   A. zanamivir vidarabine

   B. stavudine

   C. acyclovir

   D. HCl

10. When teaching a client about rifampin therapy, which of the following instructions does the nurse include?

    A. stop taking the medication if your urine turns red-orange

    B. take the medication with meals

    C. inform the health care provider if your skin starts to turn yellow

    D. take the medication with an antacid

11. Clients taking amprenavir should be instructed to take supplements of

    A. Vitamin D

    B. Vitamin C

    C. Vitamin K

    D. Vitamin E

Multiple Response

Circle the best answers for each of the following questions. More than one answer is correct.

1. When administering tetracyclines, the nurse will do which of the following? Select all that apply.

   A. Administer tetracyclines with milk.

   B. Administer tetracyclines on an empty stomach.

   C. Instruct the client to avoid excessive exposure to the sun.

   D. Avoid administration of tetracyclines to children under 8 years of age.

   E. Avoid administration of tetracyclines to women in the last two trimesters of pregnancy.

   F. Avoid administering tetracyclines simultaneously with iron preparations.

2. Which of the following will the nurse include when teaching a client who is receiving chemotherapy for tuberculosis? Select all that apply.
   A. It is common to have to take medication for the treatment of tuberculosis for almost a year.
   B. Vitamin B_6 (Pyridoxine) is used to prevent the development of peripheral neuropathy when taking isoniazid.
   C. Take rifampin with meals.
   D. Rifampin therapy may cause the urine to turn a reddish orange.
   E. Avoid use of alcohol when taking isoniazid.
   F. Clients taking para-aminosalicylic acid should take supplements of vitamin C.

3. Which of the following will the nurse include when teaching a client about zidovudine therapy? Select all that apply.
   A. If you experience a headache, take acetaminophen.
   B. Take ibuprofen to relieve muscle aches associated with use of this drug.
   C. Take this drug every 4 hours while awake.
   D. Inform the health care provider if you develop a cough.
   E. Inform the health care provider if you develop a temperature.
   F. Inform the health care provider if you have a change in your mucous membranes.

Critical Thinking Exercises

1. Discuss the procedures necessary for the safe administration of antimicrobial medications to clients.

   _____

   _____

   _____

   _____

2. Develop a method to help a client coordinate daily administration of various agents to treat infections. Include common over-the-counter medications taken on a regular basis and any precautions of which the client must be aware.

   _____

   _____

   _____

   _____

3. Present a teaching plan for clients receiving antimicrobial agents.

   _____

   _____

   _____

   _____

4. Investigate current treatment trends for tuberculosis.

   _____

   _____

   _____

   _____

5. Investigate current and proposed treatment modalities for HIV and AIDS.

   _____

   _____

   _____

   _____

CHAPTER 8 Antifungal Agents and Antiparasitic Agents

Objectives

After reading Chapter 8 of *Pharmacological Aspects of Nursing Care,* 8th edition, the student will be able to:

1. Describe clients at risk for fungal infections.
2. Discuss the mechanism of action of antifungal agents.
3. Discuss the major adverse effects associated with the use of antifungal agents.
4. Identify drug interactions associated with each antifungal agent.
5. Discuss ways in which drugs may exert antiparasitic effects.
6. Apply nursing process in the administration of antifungal and antiparasitic agents.
7. Describe nursing interventions to prevent reinfestation with parasites.
8. Successfully complete the games and activities in the online student StudyWARE.

Definitions

Supply the definitions for the following terms.

1. chloroquine _____

2. helminthiasis _____

3. amebiasis _____

4. malaria _____

5. parasites _____

6. metronidazole _____

Fill in the Blank

Write in the missing information.

1. Parasitic infections are classified as _____.
2. Malaria is caused by protozoal parasites of the genus _____.
3. The organisms responsible for the development of malaria in humans are most often inoculated by _____ but also may be transmitted by _____ or by _____.
4. Amebiasis is a parasitic disorder characterized by the invasion of the large bowel by the protozoal organism _____.
5. Chloroquine has been used for treatment of malaria as well as _____ and _____.
6. _____ is the most effective tetracycline for the treatment of *Giardia lamblia*.
7. _____ is the most common form of parasitic disease affecting humans.
8. Clients are instructed that their urine may _____ or turn _____ when taking metronidazole.

Multiple Choice

Circle the best answer for each of the following questions. There is only one answer to each question.

1. The nurse is administering chloroquine sulfate (Plaquenil) to a client. The nurse identifies this agent as useful in the treatment of malaria as well as
   A. arthritis
   B. influenza
   C. leprosy
   D. amebiasis infections

2. Clients receiving quinine should be observed for cinchonism, which is characterized by
   A. tinnitus
   B. prolonged QT interval
   C. hypertension
   D. peeling skin

3. Which of these antimalarial medications is commonly used to treat discoid lupus erythematosus?
   A. primaquine phosphate
   B. mefloquine (Lariam)
   C. chloroquine phosphate (Aralen)
   D. hydroxychloroquine (Plaquenil)

4. Nursing interventions include assessment for prolonged QT interval when the client is receiving which of the following drugs?
   A. quinine sulfate (Qualaquin)
   B. hydroxychloroquine (Plaquenil)
   C. thiaendazole (Mintezol)
   D. ivermectin (Stromectol)

5. The nurse identifies which of the following drugs as being most effective for the treatment of amebiasis?
   A. metronidazole (Flagyl)
   B. paromomycin (Humatin)
   C. halofantrine (Halfan)
   D. hydroxychloroquine (Plaquenil)

6. The nurse identifies which of the following drugs as effective in the treatment of *Pneumocystis carinii*?
   A. atovaquone (Mepron)
   B. paromomycin sulfate
   C. albendozole (Albenza)
   D. metronidazole

7. Which statement made by a new nurse teaching a client about *Trichomonas vaginalis* requires the supervising nurse to intervene?
   A. This infection is associated with a thin, yellow discharge.
   B. This infection is associated with pruritus.
   C. This infection only affects females.
   D. The discharge associated with this infection is foul smelling.

8. The most commonly diagnosed form of helminthiasis is found in humans, evidenced by
   A. red, pruritic skin
   B. serous drainage
   C. infestation with parasitic worms
   D. scabies

9. The nurse identifies which of the following agents as being effective in the treatment of onchocericiasis?
   A. ivermectin (Stromectol)
   B. praziquantel (Biltricide)
   C. thiabendazole (Mintezol)
   D. alvendazole (Albenza)

10. When providing client teaching about antimalarial drugs, which of the following does the nurse include?
    A. These medications must be taken on an empty stomach.
    B. Hypertension is the most common adverse effect of these medications.
    C. Dark-skinned persons are at a higher risk of hemolytic reactions when taking primaquine phosphate.
    D. The first signs of toxic effects of these drugs are dermatologic reactions.

Multiple Response

Circle the best answers for each of the following questions. More than one answer is correct.

1. Which of the following will the nurse include when teaching a client about antihelminic therapy? Select all that apply.

   A. Be sure to carefully cook meat before you eat it.
   B. Avoid walking barefoot.
   C. Avoid taking mebendazole with food.
   D. Swallow thiabendazole tablets whole.
   E. Adverse effects can include skin rashes.
   F. Close contacts should be examined and treated if necessary.

2. When teaching a client about metronidazole therapy, which of the following will the nurse include? Select all that apply.

   A. If your urine turns reddish brown, call the health care provider immediately.
   B. If you experience a metallic taste in your mouth, call the health care provider immediately.
   C. Avoid use of alcoholic beverages during the course of therapy.
   D. Both sexual partners need to be treated to decrease the likelihood of recurrence.
   E. This drug is safe to use during pregnancy.
   F. You should stop taking this medication when you start to feel better.

Critical Thinking Exercises

1. Discuss the procedures necessary for the safe administration of antiparasitic medications for clients and the major uses, side effects, contraindications, and routes of administration of each classification.

   _____

   _____

   _____

   _____

2. Describe each parasitic infestation and the presenting signs and symptoms of each type.

   _____

   _____

   _____

   _____

3. Discuss critical laboratory values that need to be monitored for clients receiving antimalarials and antihelmintics.

_____

_____

_____

_____

4. Discuss and compare nursing interventions for clients diagnosed with malaria, parasites, and helminthes.

_____

_____

_____

_____

CHAPTER 9 *Antiseptics and Disinfectants*

Objectives

After reading Chapter 9 of *Pharmacological Aspects of Nursing Care*, 8th edition, the student will be able to:

1. Differentiate among the uses for antiseptics, disinfectants, and germicides.
2. List the major classes of antiseptics and disinfectants and give an example of a drug from each class.
3. Describe several factors the nurse should consider in selecting an antiseptic or disinfectant for use.
4. Describe the use of urinary anti-infective agents in the treatment of urinary tract infections.
5. Apply the nursing process in the care of clients receiving urinary anti-infectives.
6. Apply the nursing process as it relates to the safe storage and effective use of antiseptics and disinfectants.
7. Discuss the most important factors in effective handwashing.
8. Successfully complete the games and activities in the online student StudyWARE.

Definitions

Supply the definitions for the following terms.

1. disinfectant _____
2. antiseptic _____
3. germicide _____
4. prophylaxis _____
5. antipruretic _____
6. effervescence _____
7. cauterize _____

Fill in the Blank

Write in the missing information.

1. _____Lysol_____ has been identified by OSHA as a possible human carcinogen and is no longer a widely used disinfectant.
2. _____Formaldehyde_____ is a disinfectant that also may be used as an embalming agent.
3. An agent commonly used to relieve throat discomfort associated with use of a nasogastric tube is _____phenol_____.
4. _____Silver nitrate_____ eye drops are no longer the first line of therapy recommended by the CDC for preventing possible eye infection in the newborn.
5. A substance used in topical hand soap products that has been indicated to have an adverse effect on aquatic life is _____triclocarban_____.
6. The most commonly used alcohol in medical procedures is _____isopropyl alcohol_____
7. _____ is no longer used as a preservative in vaccines because of its possible association with the development of autism.
8. _____Hand washing_____ has been found to be the most effective method to prevent the spread of infection.

Multiple Choice

Circle the best answer for each of the following questions. There is only one answer to each question.

1. Which action by the new nurse requires the supervising nurse to intervene? When working with hydrogen peroxide the new nurse
   A. stores the hydrogen peroxide in a cool, dark place with the lid tightly closed
   B. uses hydrogen peroxide to cleanse the inner cannula of a tracheostomy set
   C. uses hydrogen peroxide with normal saline to provide mouth care
   D. uses full strength hydrogen peroxide for wound irrigation

2. When working with isopropyl alcohol, the nurse assesses for the most common adverse effect of this agent, which is
   A. increased bleeding at incision or injection sites
   B. bleaching of the skin or hair
   C. allergic reactions
   D. darkening of the skin where the agent is used

3. Which of the following agents should the nurse use to disinfect surgical instruments?
   A. boric acid
   B. isopropanol alcohol
   C. glutaraldehyde (Cidex)
   D. provodine iodine

4. The nurse is supervising an aide who has been assigned to disinfect a surgical instrument. Which action by the aide requires the supervising nurse to intervene? The aide
   A. washes the instrument in soapy water
   B. uses friction to cleanse debris from the surgical instrument
   C. removes the instrument from the soapy water and places it in the disinfectant
   D. rinses the soap from the instrument and allows it to dry

5. The least important component of the process for effective hand hygiene is
   A. agent used
   B. frequency
   C. duration
   D. technique

6. Which of the following statements about the use of hydrogen peroxide in the care of clients does the nurse identify as true?
   A. Repeated use can cause increased scarring of wounds.
   B. The solution is very stable.
   C. Darkening of the skin occurs with use.
   D. This agent may not be used in the mouth for fear of systemic absorption and toxicity.

7. Which of the following agents does the nurse identify as first-line treatment for the care of a client with burns?
   A. provodine iodine (Betadine)
   B. salicylic acid
   C. silver nitrate
   D. silver sulfadiazine

8. Which of the following agents does the nurse identify as an effective surgical site cleanser as well as an oral rinse for gingivitis?
   A. chlorhexidine
   B. chloroxylenol
   C. benzoyl peroxide
   D. hexochlorophene

9. When teaching a family member how to care for a client with an infected wound in the home, the nurse will instruct the family member to
   A. wash contaminated linens in cool water
   B. avoid use of bleach when washing contaminated linens
   C. apply medications to the wound using firm pressure to displace tissue slightly
   D. perform hand hygiene before working with the wound

10. Which of the following statements about use of antiseptics does the nurse identify as true?

    A. Isopropanol causes vasoconstriction of blood vessels thus impairing healing.

    B. A thin layer of petroleum jelly may be used to protect healthy skin around wounds packed with Dakin's solution.

    C. When using hydrogen peroxide and saline, prepare solutions in advance for a 24-hour period.

    D. Silver nitrate may be used to decolorize skin stained by iodine preparations.

Multiple Response

Circle the best answers for each of the following questions. More than one answer is correct.

1. The CDC recommends that health care workers should wash their hands with soap and water rather than using an alcohol-based hand rub for routine decontamination in what situations? Select all that apply.

    A. if exposure to *Bacillus anthracis* is suspected or proven

    B. before eating

    C. if hands are not visibly soiled

    D. before donning sterile gloves when inserting a sterile central intravascular catheter

    E. after taking a client's blood pressure

    F. after contact with medical equipment in the immediate vicinity of the client

2. Handwashing is recommended in what situations? Select all that apply.

    A. before contact with the client

    B. after contact with the client

    C. after removing gloves

    D. after use of alcohol-based hand rub

    E. after application of nonsterile gloves

    F. before caring for another client

Critical Thinking Exercises

1. Discuss the nursing process for using antiseptics and disinfectants.

_____

_____

_____

_____

2. Review material safety data sheets from a local health care facility and share findings with the class.

_____

_____

_____

_____

3. Create a staff development poster for use of antiseptics and disinfectants in the care of clients. Focus on safety issues related to client care and staff well-being. Revise this information for use by care providers in the home.

_____

_____

_____

_____

CHAPTER 10 *Analgesic and Antipyretic Agents*

Objectives

After reading Chapter 10 of *Pharmacological Aspects of Nursing Care*, 8th edition, the student will be able to:

1. Discuss the major therapeutic actions and adverse effects of each class of analgesics and antipyretics.
2. Apply the nursing process for clients receiving each of the classes of analgesics and antipyretics.
3. Describe the gate theory of pain.
4. Apply the nursing care for a client receiving analgesic drugs via an epidural catheter.
5. Apply nursing interventions for a client receiving a placebo.
6. Describe client behaviors indicative of pain and the nursing actions that might be associated with pain control.
7. Discuss client-controlled analgesia (PCA) and identify appropriate nursing interventions for clients using PCA.
8. Successfully complete the games and activities in the online student StudyWARE.

Definitions

Supply the definitions for the following terms.

1. pain threshold _____
2. analgesic _____
3. pain tolerance _____
4. endorphins and enkephalins _____
5. euphoria _____
6. abstinence syndrome _____
7. pain _____
8. client-controlled analgesia (PCA) _____

Fill in the Blank

Write in the missing information.

1. The most popular current theory regarding pain is the *gate control theory*.

2. The neurotransmitters known as *endorphins* and *enkephalins* seem to be capable of binding with opioid receptors in the CNS, thereby inhibiting the transmission of pain impulses, producing an analgesic effect.

3. *Morphine S.* is a Schedule II controlled substance and is the prototype of opioid analgesics.

4. The gold standard therapy for the treatment of pain associated with the ischemia of acute myocardial infarction is *Morphine S.*

5. Severe respiratory depression that results from opioid use can be treated with *naloxone*.

6. *Rylomine* is an intranasal form of morphine sulfate that is currently under clinical trials.

Multiple Choice

Circle the best answer for each of the following questions. There is only one answer to each question.

1. The preferred method of administering analgesics for acute pain in the hospital setting is
   A. intravenously
   B. subcutaneously
   C. intramuscularly
   D. orally

2. Potentiation is a term that means
   A. a medication's effects will be increased when given with another medication
   B. two medications work together to provide therapeutic results
   C. the central nervous system will be depressed
   D. a medication's effects will be decreased when given with a second medication

3. The most common adverse effect of opioid analgesics is
   A. nausea
   B. constipation
   C. vomiting
   D. diarrhea

4. When administering methadone (Dolophine HCL) to a client with opioid dependence, the nurse will teach the client
   A. to avoid ingestion of any citrus juices
   B. that diarrhea is a common complication when using this drug
   C. that use of this drug will increase withdrawal symptoms
   D. that this drug has an extended duration of action

5. An opioid antagonist is given to reverse respiratory depression caused by narcotic administration. Which antagonist would commonly be prescribed?
   A. naloxone HCl
   B. hydromorphone
   C. oxycodone
   D. hydromorphone HCl

6. What is the agent of choice for the treatment of moderate to severe pain associated with postoperative visceral pain?
   A. fentanyl citrate (Sublimaze)
   B. morphine sulfate
   C. hydromorphone (Dilaudid)
   D. meperidine HCL (Demerol)

7. One of the most important considerations when deciding if a client should have a PCA pump is the client's
   A. age
   B. developmental level
   C. level of consciousness
   D. ability to understand and follow directions

8. Acute pain is defined as
   A. a duration lasting less than 6 months with one or more episodes of exacerbation
   B. pain lasting two weeks
   C. recurrent pain lasting 6 months or more
   D. pain unrelieved by the usual methods

9. A client has an epidural catheter placed for infusion of medication to treat chronic pain. The nurse will question which medication ordered to be infused via the intraspinal route?
   A. morphine sulfate
   B. hydromorphone (Dilaudid)
   C. duramorph
   D. bupivacaine

10. A client is receiving fentanyl citrate (Sublimaze) for the treatment of acute pain. It is most important for the nurse to monitor the client for
    A. nausea
    B. vomiting
    C. urticaria
    D. respiratory depression

Multiple Response

Circle the best answers for each of the following questions. More than one answer is correct.

1. Which of the following statements about morphine sulfate does the nurse identify as true? Select all that apply.
   A. It is the prototype of opioid analgesics.
   B. Use of morphine sulfate is contraindicated in the treatment of pain in children.
   C. It is effective in the treatment of pulmonary edema.
   D. The preferred method of administering morphine is by the intramuscular route.
   E. Diarrhea is the most frequent adverse effect associated with its use.
   F. It has a short half-life.

2. Which of the following statements about migraine headaches does the nurse identify as true? Select all that apply.
   A. There is usually a family history of the disease.
   B. Photophobia commonly occurs.
   C. They are a form of vascular headaches.
   D. They occur as equally severe throughout all of the head.
   E. Occurrence in childhood is rare.
   F. Clients with migraines often experience a prodromal phase.

3. Which of the following drugs does the nurse identify as opioid analgesics? Select all that apply.
   A. naltrexone HCL (Revia)
   B. pentazocine HCL (Talwin)
   C. meperidine HCL (Demerol)
   D. hydromorphone HCL (Dilaudid)
   E. fentanyl citrate (Duragesic)
   F. codeine phosphate

Critical Thinking Exercises

1. Discuss the nursing responsibilities associated with safe administration of opioid medications, as well as the necessary documentation.

   _____

   _____

   _____

   _____

2. Describe the gate theory of pain.

   _____

   _____

   _____

   _____

3. Compare and contrast nursing interventions associated with care of the client receiving nonopioid and opioid analgesics.

_____

_____

_____

_____

4. Prepare a teaching plan for client use of a PCA pump.

_____

_____

_____

_____

5. Investigate current treatment modalities for chronic pain.

_____

_____

_____

_____

6. Review current research efforts in the management of pain in end-of-life care.

_____

_____

_____

_____

CHAPTER 11 *Anesthetic Agents*

Objectives

After reading Chapter 11 of *Pharmacological Aspects of Nursing Care,* 8th edition, the student will be able to:

1. Differentiate the characteristics of the four stages of general anesthesia.
2. Discuss major therapeutic actions and adverse effects of the most commonly used preanesthetic agents.
3. Discuss major therapeutic actions and adverse effects of the most commonly used anesthetic agents.
4. Apply the nursing process for clients receiving each of the major classes of anesthetic and preanesthetic agents.
5. Discuss the client needs and appropriate nursing interventions for a client with malignant hyperthermia.
6. Successfully complete the games and activities in the online student StudyWARE.

Definitions

Supply the definitions for the following terms.

1. sedative-hypnotic _____
2. anesthetics _____
3. general anesthesia _____
4. regional anesthesia _____
5. spinal anesthesia _____
6. malignant hyperthermia _____

Fill in the Blank

Write in the missing information.

1. Anesthetics are agents that interfere with _____ and thereby diminish pain and sensation.
2. _____ block nerve conduction only in the area to which they are applied and do not cause a loss of consciousness.
3. The four stages of anesthesia are Stage 1 _____, Stage 2 _____, Stage 3 _____, and Stage 4 _____.
4. _____ is a reversible state of unconsciousness as a result of pharmacologic agents inhibiting the neuronal impulses in areas of the CNS.
5. Belladonna alkaloids are used during general anesthesia to _____, _____, and _____.
6. The first local anesthetic to be discovered was _____.
7. _____ is the drug of choice for the treatment of malignant hyperthermia.
8. To prevent headaches that follow spinal anesthesia, the client is generally kept in a recumbent position for at least _____ hours and is provided with adequate fluid replacement.

Multiple Choice

Circle the best answer for each of the following questions. There is only one answer to each question.

1. A client undergoing thoracic surgery will most likely be managed in which plane of surgical anesthesia?
   A. plane 1
   B. plane 2
   C. plane 3
   D. plane 4

2. Respiratory collapse followed by complete circulatory collapse occurs during this toxic stage of anesthesia.

   A. stage I—analgesia
   B. stage II—delirium
   C. stage III—surgical anesthesia
   D. stage IV—medullary paralysis

3. Which general anesthetic administered by inhalation is most likely to cause hepatic complications?

   A. desflurane (Suprane)
   B. enflurane (Ethrane)
   C. halothane (Fluothane)
   D. isoflurane (Forane)

4. Which of the following statements about nitrous oxide does the nurse identify as being true?

   A. It is the most popular anesthetic gas.
   B. Cylinders containing nitrous oxide are always red.
   C. Nitrous oxide is very explosive.
   D. Nitrous oxide is a very potent anesthetic.

5. The nurse identifies which of the following anesthetic agents as most often associated with the development of malignant hyperthermia?

   A. pentazocine lactate (Talwin)
   B. lidocaine (Xylocaine HCL)
   C. succinylcholine (Anectine)
   D. buprivacaine hydrochloride (Marcaine)

6. Regional anesthesia selection should be based primarily upon

   A. client preference
   B. the area to be anesthetized
   C. the cost of the agent
   D. health care provider's prior experience with the drug

7. The first action the nurse should take when the client arrives in the postanesthesia care unit (PACU) is to

   A. obtain the report from the anesthesia care provider
   B. attach the client to the cardiac monitor
   C. obtain the client's blood pressure
   D. assess the client's airway

8. Which of the following general anesthetics has a high potential for arrhythmia and should only be used if other agents are not effective?

   A. fentanyl citrate (Innovar)
   B. ketamine (Ketolar)
   C. methohexital sodium (Brevital)
   D. midazolam (Versed)

9. Promethazine hydrochloride (Phenergan) is frequently used as a sedative-hypnotic and may be combined with a reduced dose of opioid analgesic. Of what side effect should the nurses be especially aware?

   A. The medication should only be injected into large veins.
   B. It may cause discoloration of the urine, to pink or reddish brown.
   C. It may cause flushing.
   D. Protect from light to prevent precipitation.

10. The most common reaction clients experience as a result of local anesthesia is

    A. urticaria
    B. bleb formation
    C. puritis
    D. ecchymosis

11. Which of the following is an accepted finding when assessing a client receiving continuous extravascular infusion (CEI) for regional anesthesia? Client report of

    A. metallic taste
    B. blurred vision
    C. ringing in the ears
    D. pain rating of 2 on a scale of 10

12. Clients who have received ketamine hydrochloride (Ketalar) should be observed for the development of

    A. prolonged QT interval
    B. emergence delirium
    C. photosensitivity
    D. renal failure

Multiple Response

Circle the best answers for each of the following questions. More than one answer is correct

1. Before administering propofol (Diprivan) to a client, the nurse must assess the client for allergies to? Select all that apply.

   A. penicillin
   B. peanuts
   C. shellfish
   D. eggs
   E. latex
   F. soy

2. Which of the following statements about meperidine HCL (Demerol) does the nurse identify as true? Select all that apply.

   A. It is an outdated pain medication.
   B. Use of meperidine (Demerol) results in toxic metabolites.
   C. It is useful in the managment of postoperative shivering.
   D. Meperidine (Demerol) causes constipation.
   E. Meperidine (Demerol) is unsafe for use in older clients.
   F. Meperidine (Demerol) is safe to use in clients with renal failure.

3. The nurse identifies which of the following as manifestations of methemogliolanamia? Select all that apply.

   A. bradycardia
   B. pallor
   C. headache

   D. dyspnea
   E. anxiety
   F. fatigue

Critical Thinking Exercises

1. Develop a poster to summarize the changes in body function during stages and planes of anesthesia to share with members of the class. Discuss nursing responsibilities associated with each stage/plane.

   _____

   _____

   _____

   _____

2. Obtain a copy of an anesthesia flow sheet from a client's surgery and research medications documented as used for anesthesia.

   _____

   _____

   _____

   _____

3. Develop a plan of care for clients receiving general or regional anesthesia. Compare and contrast nursing responsibilities of the two.

   _____

   _____

   _____

   _____

4. Review a local health care facility's plan of prevention and treatment of malignant hyperthermia.

   _____

   _____

   _____

   _____

CHAPTER 12 *Anti-Inflammatory Agents*

Objectives

After reading Chapter 12 of *Pharmacological Aspects of Nursing Care*, 8th edition, the student will be able to:

1. Describe the mechanism of action of the nonsteroidal anti-inflammatory agents.
2. Discuss the major adverse effects and drug interactions associated with the use of nonsteroidal anti-inflammatory agents.
3. Explain the difference between the mineralcorticoid and glucocorticoid action of corticosteroids.
4. Describe the mechanism of corticosteroid action in the treatment of inflammation.
5. Discuss the major adverse effects and drug interactions associated with the use of corticosteroids.
6. Apply the nursing process to the use of steroidal and nonsteroidal anti-inflammatory agents.
7. Successfully complete the games and activities in the online student StudyWARE.

Definition

Supply the definitions for the following terms.

1. inflammation _____
2. alicylates _____
3. nonsteroidal anti-inflammatory drugs _____
4. biologic response modifiers _____
5. corticosteroids _____
6. mineralocorticoids _____
7. aspirin _____
8. prostaglandins _____
9. cortisone _____
10. COX-2 inhibitors _____

Fill in the Blank

Write in the missing information.

1. Clients taking nonsteroidal anti-inflammatory drugs are at risk for cardiovascular events such as thrombic event ___MI___, ___CVA___, and hypertension
2. If a client is allergic to ___aspirin___, client should not receive celecoxib (Celebrex).
3. Adverse effects of infliximab (Remicade) include serious infection and ↑ risk of malignancies
4. Research has shown that in addition to serious infections, the use of infliximab (Remicade) is associated with an increased evidence of herpes zoster or shingles
5. Irreversible retinal damage has been associated with the long-term use of hydroxychloroquine (Plaquenil).

Multiple Choice

Circle the best answer for each of the following questions. There is only one answer to each question.

1. A client is receiving acetylsalicylic acid (aspirin). The nurse identifies which as the most likely reason for prescribing aspirin?
   A. analgesic effect
   B. antipyretic effect
   C. inhibitory effect on platelet aggregation
   D. anti-inflammatory effect

2. A nurse is working with a client who is allergic to aspirin. The nurse should question administration of which of the following medications?

   A. acetaminophen (Tylenol)
   B. methylprednisolone (Medrol)
   C. penicillamine (Depen)
   D. celecoxib (Celebrex)

3. The nurse identifies which of the following drugs as being a COX-2 inhibitor?

   A. celecoxib (Celebrex)
   B. indomethacin (Indocin)
   C. etanercept (Enbrel)
   D. ketorolac (Toradol)

4. The nurse identifies the maximum dose of ibuprofen in a 24-hour period as

   A. 1,600 mg
   B. 2,000 mg
   C. 2,400 ng
   D. 3,200 mg

5. A client is prescribed an anti-inflammatory agent for the treatment of rheumatoid arthritis. The client asks the nurse when he can expect to experience benefits of this therapy. The best response by the nurse is

   A. 1 week
   B. 2 weeks
   C. 3 weeks
   D. 4 weeks

6. The nurse identifies the primary adverse effects associated with tumor necrosis factor drugs as

   A. renal failure
   B. electrolyte imbalance
   C. infection
   D. gastric disturbance

7. Clients receiving the antimalarial compound hydroxychloroquine must be instructed to have baseline and periodic examinations of the

   A. heart
   B. retina
   C. femur
   D. kidney

8. The nurse identifies which of the following agents as most likely to aggravate epilepsy and psychiatric disturbances?

   A. indomethacin (Indocin)
   B. ibuprofen (Motrin)
   C. piroxicam (Feldene)
   D. infliximab (Remicade)

9. Which statement should the nurse include when teaching a client about penicillamine therapy?

   A. Rotate the site of the injection of the drug.
   B. Have your vision evaluated on a regular basis.
   C. Take on an empty stomach.
   D. Avoid any foods that contain vitamin B.

10. Which statement by a client receiving long-term therapy with corticosteroids indicates further teaching is needed?

    A. "I will eat a diet that is low in sodium."
    B. "My diet will consist of foods that are low in potassium."
    C. "I will eat a high-protein diet."
    D. "I will eat a diet that is high in carbohydrates."

Multiple Response

Circle the best answers for each of the following questions. More than one answer is correct.

1. Which of the following manifestations are associated with long-term use of corticosteroids? Select all that apply.

   A. delayed healing
   B. dehydration
   C. hypoglycemia
   D. "moon face"
   E. muscle hypertrophy
   F. "buffalo hump"

2. Which of the following drugs are nonsteroidal anti-inflammatory agents? Select all that apply.

   A. adalimumab (Humira)
   B. diflunisal (Dolobid)
   C. indomethacin (Indocin)
   D. methotrexate (Rheumatrex)
   E. dexamethasone (Decadron)
   F. diclofenac (Cataflam)

Critical Thinking Exercises

1. Investigate the history of the use of salicylates in the treatment of inflammatory disorders.

   _____

   _____

   _____

   _____

2. Investigate the use of salicylates as inhibitors of platelet aggregation. Name some of the situations in which these agents are used.

   _____

   _____

   _____

   _____

3. Explain the difference between COX-1 and COX-2 inhibitors.

   _____

   _____

   _____

   _____

4. Develop a teaching plan for a client receiving biologic response modifiers for the treatment of rheumatoid arthritis.

   _____

   _____

   _____

   _____

5. Compare and contrast nursing responsibilities when caring for clients receiving short-term steroid therapy and clients receiving long-term steroid therapy.

   _____

   _____

   _____

   _____

CHAPTER 13 Agents Used to Treat Hyperuricemia and Gout

Objectives

After reading Chapter 13 of *Pharmacological Aspects of Nursing Care,* 8th edition, the student will be able to:

1. Explain the difference between primary gout and secondary gout.
2. Describe the use of cholchicine in the treatment of an acute attack of gout.
3. Contrast the mechanism(s) by which probenicid (Benemid), sulfinpyrazone (Anturane), and allopurinol (Zyloprim) reduce serum uric acid levels.
4. Describe three drugs whose action may be interfered with by probenecid (Benemid).
5. Describe three drugs whose action may be interfered with by allopurinol (Zyloprim).
6. Discuss appropriate nursing measures that would be used in the administration of allopurinol (Zyloprim), probenecid (Benemid), or sulfinpyrazone (Anturane).
7. Apply the nursing process in the care of a client with gout.
8. Successfully complete the games and activities in the online student StudyWARE.

Definitions

Supply the definitions for the following terms.

1. gout _____
2. hyperuricemia _____
3. tophi _____
4. gouty arthritis _____
5. uricosuric agent _____

Fill in the Blank

Write in the missing information.

1. Use of the drugs low dose aspirin therapy, thiazide diuretics and immunosuppressant drugs have been associated with the development of gout.
2. The highest incidence of gout is found in African American Men.
3. Uric acid is an agent formed in the body by protein breakdown.
4. The metatarsuphalangeal joint is the most susceptible to gout symptoms.
5. The most common agents used for an acute attack of gout are high doses of nonsteroidal anti-inflammatory drugs.

Multiple Choice

Circle the best answer for each of the following questions. There is only one answer to each question.

1. A client is receiving colchicine/probenicid therapy for treatment of an acute gout attack. The nurse anticipates the medication will be administered
   A. once a day
   B. every 1–2 hours
   C. every 12 hours
   D. every 8 hours

2. When administering colchicine/probenicid for an acute gout attack, the nurse needs to monitor the client for the development of which indicator that therapy needs to be terminated?
   A. tinnitus
   B. leukopenia
   C. loose stools
   D. ototoxicity

3. When assessing clients receiving medications for gout, the nurse identifies which of the following as the most common adverse effect?
   A. gastrointestinal distress
   B. tachycardia
   C. hypoglycemia
   D. bradypnea

4. Which of the following will the nurse include when teaching the client about colchicine/probenicid therapy for the treatment of gout?
   A. It is the newest drug used to treat gout.
   B. It increases the amount of uric acid the kidneys eliminate.
   C. The major side effects of the drug are nausea, vomiting, and diarrhea.
   D. Colchicine produces fewer adverse effects than nonsteroidal anti-inflammatory agents.

5. Your client is prescribed colchicine/probenicid therapy and asks you how effective this drug is for people with gouty arthritis. What is your best response?
   A. "Colchicine is successful in treating the pain of gout in about 50% of clients."
   B. "Colchicine is successful in relieving acute gouty attacks in about 90% of clients."
   C. "We really don't have any statistics on this drug, but your doctor prescribes it to all of his patients with arthritis."
   D. "It isn't as effective as nonsteroidal anti-inflammatory drugs, but this is what your doctor prefers."

6. Use of which of the following medications requires the nurse to monitor complete blood count, uric acid levels, and hepatic and renal functions?
   A. allopurinol (Zyloprim)
   B. probenecid (Benemid)
   C. naproxen (Anaprox)
   D. indomethacin (Indocin)

7. Which should the nurse include when teaching a client about use of cholchicine/probenicid for the treatment of gout?
   A. Limit the amount of fluid you drink.
   B. If you develop a headache, use aspirin.
   C. Constipation is a common complication associated with use of this drug.
   D. Notify your health care provider if you develop nausea.

8. When caring for a client on febuxostat therapy for the treatment of gout, it is most important for the nurse to assess which laboratory results?
   A. liver function
   B. renal function
   C. cholesterol levels
   D. blood glucose

9. When teaching the client about long-term use of allopurinol (Zyloprim) for the treatment of gout, the nurse will include which statement?
   A. "Allopurinol (Zyloprim) works by decreasing the inflammation associated with gout."
   B. "Drink plenty of orange juice to keep your urine acidic when taking this drug."
   C. "Report the development of a skin rash to your primary care provider."
   D. "If you experience a headache, use aspirin to treat it."

10. Which of the following drugs is used to prevent the formation of uric acid in the body?
    A. febuxostant (Uloric)
    B. probenicid
    C. sulfinpyrazone (Anturane)
    D. sulindac (Clinoril)

Multiple Response

Circle the best answers for each of the following questions. More than one answer is correct.

1. Which of the following drugs are often prescribed as continuous treatment for the prevention of recurrent attacks of gout? Select all that apply.
   A. colchicine/probenicid
   B. allopurinol (Zyloprim)
   C. naproxen (Aleve)
   D. probenicid (Benemid)
   E. sulfinpyrazone (Anturane)
   F. indomethacin (Indocin)

2. The client with gout should avoid which of the following foods high in purines? Select all that apply.

A. anchovies

B. oysters

C. shrimp

D. scallops

E. venison

F. chocolate

Critical Thinking Exercises

1. Describe the mechanism by which hyperuricemia develops in the body.

_____

_____

_____

_____

2. Explain the role of nonsteroidal anti-inflammatory drugs in the treatment of gout.

_____

_____

_____

_____

3. Research and describe the effects of colchicine and probenecid (Benemid) for use in the treatment of the client with gout.

_____

_____

_____

_____

4. Develop a teaching plan for a client who has been prescribed sulfinpyrazone (Anturane) and allopurinol (Zyloprim) for the treatment of gout.

_____

_____

_____

_____

5. Investigate what foods sold in grocery stores may be high in purines.

_____

_____

_____

_____

CHAPTER 14 *Antihistamines, Nasal Decongestants, Expectorants, and Antitussives*

Objectives

After reading Chapter 14 of *Pharmacological Aspects of Nursing Care,* 8th edition, the student will be able to:

1. Discuss the pathyphysiological changes that occur in clients with the common cold and allergic rhinitis.
2. Describe the mechanisms by which antihistamines exert their pharmacological effect.
3. Discuss five adverse effects commonly caused by antihistamines.
4. Identify three types of clients who should not use antihistamines or who should use them only with great caution.
5. Identify antihistamines that are effective in preventing or countering motion sickness, nausea, and vomiting.
6. State the mechanism by which nasal decongestants exert their pharmacological effects.
7. Describe the cause of rebound congestion.
8. Discuss five diseases in which the use of oral decongestants is contraindicated.
9. Discuss the steps for administering nasal sprays and nose drops.
10. Identify agents currently in clinical use as antitussives or expectorants.
11. State the mechanisms by which expectorant and antitussive agents exert their therapeutic effects.
12. Discuss factors to be assessed in clients taking expectorants or antitussives.
13. Discuss when the use of expectorants or antitussive agents, or both, is clinically desirable.
14. Apply the nursing process related to the administration of nasal decongestants and antihistamines.
15. Apply the nursing process to the administration of expectorant and antitussive agents.
16. Discuss factors to be assessed in persons with allergic rhinitis and the common cold.
17. Discuss three nondrug measures that can promote comfort in clients with chronic cough.
18. Successfully complete the games and activities in the online student StudyWARE.

Definitions

Supply the definitions for the following terms.

1. histamine _____
2. rebound congestion _____
3. antitussive _____
4. desensitization _____
5. fexofenadine HCL _____

Fill in the Blank

Write in the missing information.

1. _____ and _____ are conditions that collectively cause more discomfort and lost work time than all other known illnesses combined.
2. The common cold is caused by _____.
3. Irritation of the pharyngeal mucosa may also cause coughing and the development of _____.
4. In allergic rhinitis, _____ release is part of a local immunological reaction responsible for most nasal symptoms.

5. Antihistamine use is contraindicated in nursing mothers because it may _____.

6. _____ is an antihistamine that exerts a local anesthetic action that may be useful in the treatment of puritus.

7. Nasal decongestants are agents that constrict dilated blood vessels in the nasal mucosa by stimulating _____ nerve receptors in vascular smooth muscle.

8. Clients with _____, _____, or _____ should be cautioned that some antihistamines and decongestants can aggravate these conditions.

Multiple Choice

Circle the best answer for each of the following questions. There is only one answer to each question.

1. Which of the following medications may be used as a sedative, antiemetic, and adjunct to analgesics?
   - A. beclomethasone (Vancenase)
   - B. fexofenadine HCL (Allegra)
   - C. promethazine HCl (Phenergan)
   - D. pseudoephedrine (Sudafed)

2. The nurse teaches the client that allergic rhinitis is
   - A. an immunological response caused by allergens contacting the nasal mucosa
   - B. a result of bacterial-induced injury
   - C. a condition caused by a virus
   - D. pharyngeal irritation

3. Which of the following antihistamines is used primarily for the treatment of motion sickness and vertigo?
   - A. HCL (Zyrtec)
   - B. clemastine fumarate (Tavist)
   - C. meclizine HCL (Antivert)
   - D. loratadine (Claritin)

4. Which complication with use of dimenhydrinate HCL (Dramamine) therapy should the nurse assess for?
   - A. cardiac toxicity
   - B. somnolence
   - C. anemia
   - D. masking ototoxicity of other drugs

5. When working with young children, the nurse should administer topical decongestants how many minutes prior to feedings to facilitate breathing during sucking or eating?
   - A. 15
   - B. 30
   - C. 20
   - D. 45

6. Which of the following medications does the nurse identify as an intranasal steroid product?
   - A. phenylephrine HCL (Neo-Synephrine)
   - B. dexchlorpheniramine maleate (Mylaramine)
   - C. fluticasone propionate
   - D. pseudoephedrine sulfate (Afrin)

7. The nurse will exert extreme caution when administering decongestants and antihistamines to a client with
   - A. narrow-angle glaucoma
   - B. respiratory infections
   - C. sinusitis
   - D. allergic rhinitis

8. Which of the following medications may be used for the treatment of Parkinson's disease?
   - A. ephedrine (Adrenalin)
   - B. oxymetazoline HCL (Afrin)
   - C. diphenhydramine HCl (Benadryl)
   - D. budesonide (Rhinocort)

9. Which of the following antihistamines does not cause drowsiness?
   - A. dexchlorpheniramine maleate (Mylaramine)
   - B. cetirizine hydrochloride (Zyrtec)
   - C. clemastine fumarate (Tavist)
   - D. dimenhydrinate HCL (Dramamine)

10. The nurse should question a drug order for levocetirizine dihydrochloride (Xyzal) for a client with a history of
    - A. liver disease
    - B. kidney disease
    - C. hypertension
    - D. diabetes mellitus

Multiple Response

Circle the best answers for each of the following questions. More than one answer is correct.

1. The nurse understands that use of oral decongestant drugs is contraindicated for clients with which of the following? Select all that apply.
   - A. hypertension
   - B. heart disease
   - C. diabetes mellitus
   - D. hypothyroidism
   - E. renal failure
   - F. rheumatoid arthritis

2. The nurse should instruct clients with hypertension, glaucoma, and prostate disease that the following medications may aggravate these conditions. Select all that apply.
   - A. beclomethasone dipropionate (Beconase)
   - B. budesonide (Rhinocort)
   - C. pseudoephedrine HCL (Sudafed)
   - D. epinephrine HCL (Adrenalin Chloride)
   - E. phenylephrine HCL (Neo-Synephrine)
   - F. oxymetazoline HCL (Afrin)

Critical Thinking Exercises

1. Describe the effect of the release of histamine in the body in response to tissue damage and the presence of microorganisms and allergens invading body tissues.

2. Compare the use of antihistamines in the treatment of the common cold and in allergic rhinitis.

3. Create a teaching plan for a client taking antihistamine medications, including interventions and ways to maintain client safety.

4. Develop a teaching plan for a client taking decongestants and intranasal steroid products.

5. Describe the correct techniques for self-administration of nasal spray, administration of nose drops, and use of nasal inhaler.

_____

_____

_____

_____

CHAPTER 15 *Bronchodilators and Other Respiratory Agents*

Objectives

After reading Chapter 15 of *Pharmacological Aspects of Nursing Care,* 8th edition, the student will be able to:

1. Explain the mechanism by which adrenergic stimulants and xanthine derivatives produce bronchodilation.
2. Discuss four adverse effects commonly seen in the use of bronchodilator agents.
3. Discuss factors to be assessed in persons with chronic obstructive pulmonary disease (COPD).
4. Discuss medications used to treat cystic fibrosis.
5. Explain how agents are used in the treatment of pulmonary hypertension.
6. Apply nursing interventions appropriate in the administration of bronchodilator and mucolytic agents.
7. Discuss the mechanism by which cromolyn sodium and beclomethasone diproprinate act in preventing asthmatic attacks.
8. Discuss the appropriate method of administration, adverse effects, and nursing actions used in the administration of cromolyn sodium and beclomethasone diproprinate.
9. List four nondrug methods by which ease of breathing can be promoted in a client with COPD.
10. Describe the proper method of using an oral inhaler.
11. Apply the nursing process in the care of clients with lower respiratory conditions.
12. Successfully complete the games and activities in the online student StudyWARE.

Definitions

Supply the definitions for the following terms.

1. chronic obstructive pulmonary disease (COPD) _____
2. zafirlukast _____
3. beractant _____
4. status asthmaticus _____
5. acetylcysteine _____
6. cromolyn sodium (Intal) _____
7. omalizomba (Xolair) _____
8. mucolytic _____

Fill in the Blank

Write in the missing information.

1. Leukotrienes contribute to the development of _____, _____, and _____.
2. When administering acetylcysteine, it is important to avoid contact with _____, _____, and _____.
3. The therapeutic serum level of theophylline is _____ mcg/mL.
4. Clients on sympathomimetics should not use _____ as these agents may potentiate sympathomimetic activity and cause hypertensive crisis.
5. Two examples of Leukotriene receptor antagonists include _____ and _____.
6. Common adverse effects of bronchodilators include _____, _____, and _____.

Multiple Choice

Circle the best answer for each of the following questions. There is only one answer to each question.

1. When assessing a client who has overdosed on albuterol, the nurse is most likely to find the client exhibiting

   A. bronchodilation and tachycardia
   B. bradycardia and tachypnea
   C. tachycardia and bronchoconstriction
   D. visual changes and palpitations

2. The nurse is responsible to obtain theophylline levels for a client. The optimal times for blood draws are

   A. 3 hours after immediate-release medication, 4 hours after sustained-release medication
   B. 1–2 hours after immediate-release medication, 4 hours after sustained-release medication
   C. 4 hours after immediate-release medication, 6 hours after sustained-release medication
   D. 2 hours after immediate-release medication, 6 hours after sustained-release medication

3. A client receiving a sympathomimetic agent has the following drugs ordered. Which drug order should the nurse question?

   A. tricyclic antidepressants
   B. monoamine oxidase inhibitor
   C. acetylcholinesterase
   D. prazosin

4. When caring for clients with COPD who do not have cardiac or renal health problems, how much fluid should the client receive daily?

   A. 1,200–1,800 mL
   B. 1,800–2,500 mL
   C. 2,000–3,000 mL
   D. 3,000–4,000 mL

5. The supervising nurse should intervene when he observes a new nurse caring for a patient with COPD

   A. administer high levels of oxygen for dyspnic episodes
   B. keep the head of the bed elevated
   C. administer bronchodilators in the morning
   D. administer theophylline with food

6. Which medication is contraindicated in the treatment of a client with COPD who also has a history of glaucoma?

   A. theophylline (Theolair)
   B. ipratropium bromide (Atrovent)
   C. tiotropium bromide (Spiriva)
   D. zileuton (Zyflo)

7. Which statement by a parent whose neonate is being treated with beractant (Survanta) indicates that more teaching is indicated?

   A. "This medication is administered intravenously."
   B. "It is used for the treatment of asthma in babies."
   C. "This medication is a natural lung surfactant derived from the lungs of animals."
   D. "The medication needs to be administered every 2 hours for 24 hours."

8. Which medication is indicated in the treatment of an acute asthma attack?

   A. cromolyn sodium (Intal)
   B. omalizumab (Xolair)
   C. zileuton (Zyflo)
   D. epinephrine (Primatene)

9. The nurse identifies the action of sympathomimetic drugs as

   A. promoting cyclic adenosine momophosphate (cAMP) production
   B. inhibiting AMP destruction by phosphodiesterase
   C. antagonizing the leukotriene-mediated bronchoconstriction associated with asthma
   D. antagonizing the action of acetylcholine

10. The nurse identifies the primary use of nedrocromil sodium (Tilade) as a treatment for

    A. respiratory distress syndrome
    B. emphysema
    C. itching associated with allergic conjunctivitis
    D. reduction of thickness and stickiness of pulmonary secretions

Multiple Response

Circle the best answers for each of the following questions. More than one answer is correct.

1. Which of the following will the nurse include when teaching a client proper use of an oral inhaler? Select all that apply.

   A. Shake the inhaler before use.
   B. Insert the metal stem of the inhaler on the flattened portion of the mouthpiece.
   C. Open the mouth and place the mouthpiece just past the lips.
   D. Push the cylinder down twice and inhale rapidly.
   E. Remove the mouthpiece and hold breath for several seconds.
   F. Exhale slowly for several seconds.

2. Which of the following statements will the nurse include when teaching a client about the management of COPD? Select all that apply.

   A. When taking sympathomimetics, avoid the use of levothyroxine sodium.
   B. Clients taking xanthines are at risk for the development of hyperkalemia.
   C. The muscle should be massaged after injection of epinephrine.
   D. Xanthines have been found to depress the CNS.
   E. Clients with liver disease should avoid use of zileuton (Zyflo).
   F. Mucolytics are usually administered by nebulization.

Critical Thinking Exercises

1. Compare and contrast the mechanism of action and adverse effects of sympathomimetic agents and xanthime bronchodilators and summarize appropriate client teaching for use of these agents.

   _____

   _____

   _____

   _____

2. Develop a graphic representation of the action of leukotriene receptor antagonists and 5-lipoxygenase inhibitors in the treatment of clients with asthma.

   _____

   _____

   _____

   _____

3. Develop a teaching plan for use of mucolytics for a client who has a longstanding history of chronic bronchitis, osteoarthritis of the hands and feet, and impaired vision as a result of macular degeneration.

   _____

   _____

   _____

   _____

4. Develop a plan of care for a client with asthma, and compare similarities and differences for the care of a client with emphysema.

_____

_____

_____

_____

CHAPTER 16 *Antiarrhythmic Agents: Cardiac Stimulants and Depressants*

Objectives

After reading Chapter 16 of *Pharmacological Aspects of Nursing Care,* 8th edition, the student will be able to:

1. Distinguish between positive and negative inotropic effects, positive and negative chronotropic effects, and positive and negative dromotropic effects of agents on the heart.

2. Discuss the mechanisms by which cardiac glycosides provide effective treatment for heart failure.

3. Discuss three factors affecting the selection of an appropriate cardiac glycoside for a particular client.

4. Define a digitalizing dose.

5. Discuss the most common gastrointestinal, neurological, and cardiac adverse effects indicative of cardiac glycoside intoxication.

6. Discuss three factors that may predispose a client to the development of cardiac glycoside toxicity.

7. Describe the mechanism of action and adverse effects related to the use of calcium-channel blocking agents.

8. Describe three ways in which antiarrhythmic drugs act to diminish or obliterate rhythm disturbances of the heart.

9. Discuss the most common adverse effects and drug interactions associated with antiarrhythmic agents.

10. Discuss the mechanism of action and common adverse effects of the cardiac stimulants most commonly used in the treatment of shock.

11. Apply the nursing process for clients receiving cardiac drugs.

12. Successfully complete the games and activities in the online student StudyWARE.

Definitions

Supply the definitions for the following terms.

1. digoxin _____

2. positive inotropic effect _____

3. negative inotropic effect _____

4. positive chronotropic effect _____

5. negative chronotropic effect _____

6. positive dromotropic effect _____

7. antiarrhythmic medications _____

8. sinoatrial (SA) node _____

9. atrioventricular (AV) node _____

10. automaticity _____

Fill in the Blank

Write in the missing information.

1. Cardiac glycosides and digoxin inhibit _____, an enzyme that regulates the amount of sodium and potassium in the cell.

2. An increase of free calcium within the cell increases the amount of _____, which is a major protein responsible for muscle contraction.

3. _____ has evolved as the most popular cardiac glycoside in the United States.

4. Normal digoxin levels are _____ ng/mL.

5. _____ classification is a system that describes drugs used to treat arrhythmias.

6. _____ is the drug of choice to treat premature ventricular contractions (PVC), particularly those following an acute myocardial infarction.

7. _____ has been used for decades for the treatment of convulsive disorders and has been found to be particularly effective in the treatment of arrhythmias caused by cardiac glycoside intoxication.

8. Diltiazem (Cardizem) is administered intravenously to treat arrhythmias and orally to treat _____.

9. Cardiac glycosides should not be administered with _____.

10. Clients taking amiodarone therapy should be assessed for the development of _____.

Multiple Choice

Circle the best answer for each of the following questions. There is only one answer to each question.

1. A client is experiencing premature ventricular contractions after a myocardial infarction. Which drug does the nurse identify as most effective in the treatment of this client?

   A. procanimide HCl

   B. phenytoin sodium

   C. lidocaine HCl

   D. bretylium tosylate

2. The nurse is particularly concerned about the development of pulmonary toxicity if a client is taking which of the following drugs?

   A. verapamil HCl

   B. diltiazem HCl

   C. esmolol HDl

   D. amiodarone HCl

3. Use of bretylium tosylate is contraindicated in the treatment of clients who have a history of

   A. diabetes mellitus

   B. lymphoma

   C. aortic stenosis

   D. chronic obstructive pulmonary disease

4. Which of the following symptoms will most likely be reported by the client who has cardiac glycoside toxicity?

   A. central nervous system (CNS) depression

   B. respiratory depression

   C. yellow or green-tinted vision

   D. constipation

5. When working with clients receiving drugs to treat arrhythmias, the nurse should be concerned about which common adverse effect of this treatment?

   A. arrhythmias

   B. hypoglycemia

   C. rash

   D. hepatic failure

6. Which of the following statements by a client indicates that more teaching about digoxin therapy is indicated?

   A. "I will take an antacid with digoxin to prevent stomach upset."

   B. "I will call the health care provider if my pulse rate is below 60 beats per minute."

   C. "I will call the health care provider if the color of my vision changes."

   D. "I will follow up with my health care provider at routine intervals."

7. A client's digoxin serum level is 3.5 ng/mL. The first action by the nurse should be to

   A. assess vital signs

   B. notify the health care provider

   C. raise the head of the client's bed

   D. administer oxygen

8. Oxytocic drugs, when used concurrently with adrenergic stimulants in obstetric clients to correct hypotension, may cause complications. It is most important for the nurse to monitor the client for

   A. life-threatening arrhythmias

   B. peripheral vasoconstriction

   C. sympathomimetic response

   D. hypertension, resulting in cerebral blood vessel rupture postpartum

9. The nurse should teach the client receiving mexiletine (Mexitil) to avoid which of the following in his or her diet?
   A. nuts
   B. bananas
   C. cranberry juice
   D. lunch meats

10. The nurse identifies which of the following drugs as most effective in the treatment of supraventricular tachycardia?
   A. lidocaine
   B. flecainide acetate
   C. procainamide HDl
   D. verapamil HCl

11. Before the administration of each dose of cardiac glycoside medication is given, the nurse should
   A. check the radial pulse for 30 seconds
   B. check the apical pulse for one full minute
   C. hold the medication if the client's heart rate is 60 bpm
   D. check the client's serum digoxin level

12. Which of the following statements about lidocaine does the nurse identify as being true?
   A. It is predominantly metabolized in the kidney.
   B. It is ineffective if administered orally.
   C. It commonly causes hypertension as an adverse effect.
   D. It slows the rate of conduction of electrical impulses in the heart.

Multiple Response

Circle the best answers for each of the following questions. More than one answer is correct.

1. The nurse identifies which of the following as the most common adverse effects of cardiac glycoside therapy? Select all that apply.
   A. constipation
   B. halo vision
   C. ambylopia
   D. bradycardia
   E. bigeminal rhythm
   F. diplopia

2. Which of the following statements about milrinone (Primacor) does the nurse identify as being true? Select all that apply.
   A. It exerts a negative inotropic effect.
   B. It causes vasoconstriction.
   C. It is used for the short-term management of heart failure.
   D. The drug should be diluted in dextrose solution before administration.
   E. Do not administer furosemide (Lasix) with this drug.
   F. It may cause arrhythmias.

Critical Thinking Exercises

1. Develop a display that shows the flow of electrical impulses through the heart and identify where and how each drug used to treat arrhythmias exerts its therapeutic effect.

_____

_____

_____

_____

2. Review the history of the use of cardiac glycosides.

_____

_____

_____

_____

3. Review the methods used to determine correct dosing for clients receiving cardiac glycosides.

_____

_____

_____

_____

4. Develop a teaching plan for a client taking cardiac glycosides.

_____

_____

_____

_____

5. Make a chart summarizing the action and nursing responsibilities associated with drugs in the Vaughan Williams classification system.

_____

_____

_____

_____

6. Describe nursing responsibilities associated with the use of cardiac stimulants to treat shock.

_____

_____

_____

_____

CHAPTER 17 *Agents That Dilate Coronary Blood Vessels*

Objectives

After reading Chapter 17 of *Pharmacological Aspects of Nursing Care,* 8th edition, the student will be able to:

1. Discuss two theories that may explain how nitrates reduce anginal pain.
2. Identify the common routes of nitroglycerin administration and the advantages associated with each.
3. Explain the storage requirements necessary for nitroglycerin tablets to retain their potency.
4. Discuss methods of minimizing the development of tolerance and of producing renewed sensitivity to the action of nitrates and nitrites.
5. Discuss the major adverse effects associated with the use of nitrates.
6. Describe the procedures to be used in the administration of amyl nitrite and topically applied nitroglycerin products.
7. Apply the nursing process related to caring for clients receiving coronary vasodilators.
8. Successfully complete the games and activities in the online student StudyWARE.

Definitions

Supply the definitions for the following terms.

1. nitrate-induced headache _____
2. atenolol (Tenormin) _____
3. acute myocardial infarction (AMI) _____
4. nicardipine (Cardene) _____
5. isosorbide dinitrate (Isordil) _____

Fill in the Blank

Write in the missing information.

1. _____ has traditionally been the drug most often used in the symptomatic relief of angina.
2. Because of their beta-adrenergic blocking action, beta-adrenergic blocking agents are contraindicated for use in clients with _____, _____, _____, _____, _____, or _____.
3. When used with nitrates, beta-adrenergic blocking agents may increase the chance of the client developing the adverse effect of _____.
4. Among the first drugs to be administered in the event of an acute myocardial infarction is _____ followed by _____.
5. A fresh supply of nitroglycerine should be obtained by the client every _____ months.
6. Nitroglycerine for intravenous administration must be diluted in _____ or _____.

Multiple Choice

Circle the best answer for each of the following questions. There is only one answer to each question.

1. The number one cause of death in the United States is
   A. ischemic heart disease
   B. stroke
   C. breast cancer
   D. lung cancer

2. Clients with Prinzmetal's angina are most often treated with

   A. calcium-channel blockers
   B. beta-adrenergic blockers
   C. nitrates
   D. anticoagulants

3. Nitroglycerin, given sublingually, usually relieves anginal chest pain within _____ minutes in 90% of clients.

   A. 10
   B. 15
   C. 5
   D. 1

4. A client is prescribed a beta-adrenergic agent and a nitrate for treatment of angina pectoris. The nurse will instruct the client to

   A. take the beta-adrenergic blocker before the nitrate
   B. take the beta-blocker on an empty stomach, then take the nitrate 2 hours later
   C. take the medications together
   D. expect to experience a change in urine color as a result of this therapy

5. A new nurse is preparing to administer nitroglycerine intravenously. Which of the following actions by the nurse requires the supervising nurse to intervene? The new nurse

   A. dilutes the nitroglycerine with 5% dextrose
   B. infuses the nitroglycerine with a piggyback antibiotic
   C. uses an infusion pump to administer the medication
   D. dilutes the nitroglycerine with 0.9% sodium chloride

6. Which of the following statements by a client indicates that more teaching about transdermal nitroglycerine is needed?

   A. I will remove all of the previous medication before applying the new medication.
   B. I will apply the medication to a hairless part of my upper body.
   C. I will change the application site daily.
   D. I will store the medication in the refrigerator.

7. When teaching a client about sublingual nitroglycerine, the nurse will include which of the following?

   A. Obtain a fresh supply every 3 months.
   B. A slight burning sensation when the product is used indicates that the product is fresh.
   C. Carry a container of the medication next to your body.
   D. Keep a cotton ball in with the tablets to prevent them from moving.

8. When administering nitroglycerine intravenously, the nurse must

   A. infuse the nitroglycerine through central venous access
   B. dilute the nitroglycerine with Ringer's Lactate only to hemodynamically stable clients
   C. use an infusion pump
   D. using reinforced plastic containers

9. Prinzmetal's angina is defined as

   A. anginal pain occurring when patient is at rest
   B. a result of closure of the coronary artery with plaque
   C. the first phase of an acute myocardial infarction
   D. anginal pain that only occurs early in the morning

10. When working with a client receiving transdermal nitroglycerine, the nurse will teach the client to

    A. remove the previous transdermal system after applying the current transdermal system
    B. rise slowly from a sitting or lying position
    C. apply the transdermal system before the first meal of the day
    D. identify a burning sensation in the mouth as a positive sign of drug potency

Multiple Response

Circle the best answers for each of the following questions. More than one answer is correct.

1. Which of the following does the nurse identify as true in the treatment of the client with a myocardial infarction? Select all that apply.

   A. Aspirin is administered to break up clots that have formed.
   B. Morphine is used to cause coronary artery vasodilation and produce analgesia.
   C. Nitroglycerine is administered to decrease the heart's workload.
   D. Beta blockers are used to increase the heart rate.
   E. ACE inhibitors are used to help reduce the risk for death or congestive heart failure.
   F. Calcium-channel blockers are used to decrease oxygen supply.

2. When applying nitroglycerine via a transdermal system, the nurse will do which of the following? Select all that apply.

   A. Take the client's blood pressure.
   B. Remove the previously applied dose.
   C. Put on gloves.
   D. Place the transdermal system on the same site as the previous dose.
   E. Rub the transdermal system into the skin.
   F. Check the client's blood pressure 5 minutes after the medication is applied.

3. When teaching the client about the use of nitrates, which of the following will the nurse include? Select all that apply.

   A. Discard unused sublingual tablets 6 months after opening the original bottle.
   B. Chew tablets thoroughly before swallowing them.
   C. If chest pain develops, stop any activity, rest, and take 1 nitroglycerine tablet.
   D. You may take up to 5 tablets in 5 minutes if you have chest pain.
   E. If chest pain continues after the second tablet, call 911.
   F. The occurrence of headache usually decreases with increasing use.

Critical Thinking Exercises

1. Describe the use of nitrates in the treatment of angina.

   _____

   _____

   _____

   _____

2. Compare and contrast the nursing responsibilities associated with treatment of the client with angina pectoris using beta-adrenergic blockers and calcium-channel blockers.

   _____

   _____

   _____

   _____

3. Develop a teaching plan for use with a client and one for professional health care providers on the appropriate method for working with transdermal nitroglycerine.

   _____

   _____

   _____

   _____

CHAPTER 18 *Diuretics and Antihypertensives*

Objectives

After reading Chapter 18 of *Pharmacological Aspects of Nursing Care,* 8th edition, the student will be able to:

1. Discuss the major health conditions for which treatment with diuretic drugs is used.
2. Discuss the primary use of classes of diuretics, their mechanism of action, their adverse effects, and their drug interactions.
3. Explain the mechanism of action and major adverse effects for each of the commonly used antihypertensive drugs.
4. Discuss major nursing diagnoses and goals in caring for clients with hypertension.
5. Discuss the role of dietary sodium in preventing and controlling hypertension.
6. Describe two ways in which the nurse can increase client cooperation with a hypertension treatment plan.
7. Discuss specific ways in which the nurse can minimize the adverse effects of antihypertensive drug therapy.
8. Discuss the long-term management of hypertensive clients.
9. Apply the nursing process when caring for a client experiencing hypertension.
10. Apply the nursing process when caring for a client experiencing a hypertensive emergency.
11. Successfully complete the games and activities in the online student StudyWARE.

Definitions

Supply the definitions for the following terms.

1. thiazide diuretics _____
2. osmotic diuretics _____
3. hypertension _____
4. angiotensin-converting enzyme inhibitors _____
5. calcium-channel blocking agents _____

Fill in the Blank

Write in the missing information.

1. When thiazide diuretics are used for prolonged periods of time, it is often necessary to provide _____ and _____ supplementation.
2. Along with electrolyte imbalances, the use of loop diuretics administered parenterally in high doses has been associated with _____.
3. Normal blood pressure is defined as _____ systolic over _____ diastolic.
4. The DASH diet acronym stands for _____ _____ to _____ _____.
5. Medications used in the treatment of hypertensive emergencies include _____, _____, and _____.

Multiple Choice

Circle the best answer for each of the following questions. There is only one answer to each question.

1. When working with clients receiving thiazide diuretics, the nurse anticipates the need for the client to have supplementation with

    A. sodium

    B. calcium

    C. potassium

    D. magnesium

2. The nurse identifies which of the following medications as most likely to cause excessive growth of fine body hair during therapy?

    A. amlodipine

    B. betaxolol

    C. benazepril HCl

    D. minoxidil

3. Which of the following does the nurse identify as a potassium-sparing diuretic?

    A. spironolactone

    B. hydrochlorothiazide

    C. furosemide

    D. atenolol

4. When administering medamylamine HCl therapy to a client, it is important for the nurse to asses for which adverse effects?

    A. ileus

    B. asthma

    C. low platelet counts

    D. hypertension

5. Which of the following medications does the nurse anticipate for use in the treatment of hypertensive emergencies?

    A. acetazolamide

    B. methazolamide

    C. labetolol

    D. propanolol

6. A new nurse is administering nitroprusside sodium. Which action by the nurse requires the supervising nurse to intervene? The new nurse

    A. protects the solution from light

    B. dissolves the nitroprusside in D5W

    C. monitors the client for cyanide toxicity

    D. assesses the client's blood pressure every hour

7. Which statement by a client receiving nicardipine therapy indicates that more teaching is indicated?

    A. "I will take this medication with grapefruit juice."

    B. "I will get up slowly from a seated position."

    C. "I will have my blood pressure checked on a regular basis."

    D. "I will take this medication at the same time every day."

8. The nurse identifies which of the following medications as causing dry cough as an adverse effect of therapy?

    A. benazepril HCl

    B. captopril

    C. felodipine

    D. bumetanide

9. The nurse identifies which of the following as the most common symptom associated with hypertension?

    A. diarrhea

    B. insomnia

    C. constipation

    D. headache

10. When administering bumetanide therapy to a client, it is most important for the nurse to monitor which of the following laboratory values?

    A. sodium

    B. potassium

    C. magnesium

    D. bicarbonate

Multiple Response

Circle the best answers for each of the following questions. More than one answer is correct.

1. While the nurse is assessing a client's blood pressure at a wellness fair, the result is abnormally high. The nurse will do which of the following? Select all that apply.

    A. Immediately retake the blood pressure and compare findings.
    B. Retake the blood pressure with a cuff one size larger and compare findings.
    C. Ask the client to follow up with his or her health care provider in 1 week.
    D. Wait 10 minutes to retake the blood pressure.
    E. Retake the blood pressure in 10 minutes and if it is still above the normal range refer the client to his or her health care provider.
    F. Ask the client if he or she is taking any medications.

2. Which of the following will the nurse include when teaching a client about medication therapy for the management of hypertension? Select all that apply.

    A. If erectile dysfunction occurs while taking the medication, stop taking it immediately.
    B. If you have diabetes mellitus and are taking beta blockers, you are at high risk for the development of hyperglycemia.
    C. You should get up slowly from a seated position.
    D. If you have nasal congestion, avoid use of over-the-counter nasal decongestants.
    E. If you have diabetes mellitus and take a thiazide diuretic, you need to be aware than you may develop hyperglycemia.
    F. Report any muscle weakness, leg cramps, or pulse irregularities as these may indicate a low potassium level.

Critical Thinking Exercises

1. Explore the use of diuretics and antihypertesives in the treatment of hypertension. How are they similar in action and how do they differ?

    _____

    _____

    _____

    _____

2. Develop a teaching plan for a client taking each of the following diuretics: thiazide, loop, potassium-sparing, osmotic, carbonic anhydrase inhibitors, and combination potassium-sparing and hydrochlorothiazide diuretics. Focus on client safety issues when taking these medications.

    _____

    _____

    _____

    _____

3. Compare and contrast nursing responsibilities to clients associated with the administration of nondiuretic antihypertensive medications.

    _____

    _____

    _____

    _____

4. Develop a client teaching plan for long-term management of hypertension using antihypertensive medications. Focus on client safety issues.

_____

_____

_____

_____

CHAPTER 19 *Agents Used to Treat Hyperlipidemia*

Objectives

After reading Chapter 19 of *Pharmacological Aspects of Nursing Care,* 8th edition, the student will be able to:

1. Discuss the major risk factors associated with the development of atherosclerosis.
2. Explain the mechanism of action of each class of agents used in the treatment of hyperlipidemia.
3. Discuss the role of diet and drug therapies in the control of hyperlipidemia.
4. Discuss the common adverse effects of agents used to treat hyperlipidemia.
5. Select the proper method of administering agents commonly used for the treatment of hyperlipidemia.
6. Explain significant drug interactions associated with drugs used in the treatment of hyperlipidemia.
7. Apply the nursing process related to the administration of agents used to treat hyperlipidemia.
8. Discuss common factors to be included in a comprehensive nursing assessment of the client with hyperlipidemia.
9. Successfully complete the games and activities in the online student StudyWARE.

Definitions

Supply the definitions for the following terms.

1. atherosclerosis _____
2. high-density lipoproteins (HDL) _____
3. low-density lipoproteins (LDL) _____
4. very low-density lipoproteins (VLDL) _____
5. chylomicrons _____
6. HMG-CoA reductase inhibitors _____

Fill in the Blank

Write in the missing information.

1. It has been determined that _____ and _____ play the most important roles in promoting the development of atherosclerosis.
2. The newest class of antihyperlipidemic drugs is the _____.
3. Total cholesterol should be less than_____mg/dL, LDL should be less than _____ mg/dL, triglycerides should be less than _____ mg/dL, and HDL levels should be greater than _____ mg/dL.
4. _____ is a breakdown of muscle tissue that sometimes results from HMG-CoA inhibitor therapy.
5. Nondrug therapies for the treatment of hyperlipidemia include _____, _____, and _____.

Multiple Choice

Circle the best answer for each of the following questions. There is only one answer to each question.

1. When monitoring for adverse effects of simbastatin (Zocor), it is most important for the nurse to monitor for

   A. hypolipidemia
   B. the lowering of low-density lipoprotein (LDL) levels
   C. hepatic functional changes
   D. the raising of high-density lipoprotein (HDL) levels

2. Which of the following medications increases, or does not change, triglyceride levels?

   A. cholestyramine
   B. fluvastatin

   C. nicotinic acid
   D. rosuvastatin

3. Which of the following medications must be used with extreme caution in clients with extensive histories of alcohol consumption or liver disease?

   A. gemfibrozil (Lopid)
   B. cholestyramine (Questran)

   C. simbastatin (Zocor)
   D. nicotinic acid (Niacin)

4. When teaching a client about laboratory values and the treatment of hyperlipidemia, which will be included?

   A. Total cholesterol of 220 mg/dL is normal
   B. LDL of of 150 mg/dL is normal

   C. Triglyceride of 200 mg/dL is normal
   D. HDL of 50 mg/dL is normal

5. When administering bile sequesterants to the client, the nurse will

   A. administer powders in dry form
   B. administer bile sequestrants with other oral medications
   C. assess the client for adverse reactions of the gastrointestinal tract
   D. teach the client that the medication works by increasing the amount of cholesterol excreted by the kidney

6. Clients taking nicotinic acid often complain of flushing and pruritus. Which medication is commonly prescribed to help relieve these symptoms?

   A. gemfibrozil
   B. acetaminophen

   C. acetylsalicylic acid
   D. sodium nitroprusside

7. The nurse should teach the client receiving HMG-CoA reductase inhibitors to immediately report which of the following conditions to the health care provider?

   A. hyperalertness
   B. constipation

   C. diarrhea
   D. unexplained muscle pain

8. The nurse will instruct the client to take HMG-CoA reductase inhibitor at what time?

   A. 900
   B. 1200

   C. 1400
   D. 2000

9. The nurse identifies the most serious side effect of long-term use of exchange resins as

   A. hypoprothrombinemia
   B. elevated chloride levels

   C. hemorrhoids
   D. vitamin A deficiency

10. Which of the following statements by the client receiving treatment for hyperlipidemia indicates that more teaching is necessary?

    A. "I need to take the medications even when I feel well."
    B. "I will most likely take the medications for 2 weeks and then be able to stop."
    C. "I should also limit the amount of saturated fats in my diet."
    D. "I will increase the amount of fluids I drink every day."

Multiple Response

Circle the best answers for each of the following questions. More than one answer is correct.

1. Which of the following laboratory values does the nurse identify as being abnormal? Select all that apply.

   A. HDL 30 mg/dL
   B. total cholesterol 180 mg/dL
   C. triglyceride 160 mg/dL

   D. LDL 90 mg/dL
   E. potassium 4.0 mEq/L
   F. sodium 140 mEq/L

2. The nurse identifies which of the following statements about HMG-CoA reductase inhibitors as being true? Select all that apply.

   A. Research indicates that older adults may not live longer as a result of lowering serum cholesterol levels.

   B. Painful muscle conditions associated with administration of HMG-CoA reductase inhibitors may result in renal failure.

   C. These agents should be administered with the client's breakfast.

   D. Liver function tests should be performed before clients start therapy with these agents.

   E. Clients using these agents should be informed that photosensitivity may occur.

   F. All of the drugs in this class are contraindicated during pregnancy.

Critical Thinking Exercises

1. Discuss the types of agents used for hyperlipidemia, and describe their effects and contraindications.

2. Create a teaching plan for a client taking antihyperlipidemic agents. Specify techniques for promoting client safety.

3. Develop a chart describing the mechanism of action of HMG-CoA reductase inhibitors, fibrates, nicotinic acid, and bile sequestrants.

4. Develop a diet plan for clients who are trying to lower their cholesterol.

CHAPTER 20 Agents Affecting Blood Clotting

Objectives

After reading Chapter 20 of *Pharmacological Aspects of Nursing Care,* 8th edition, the student will be able to:

1. Discuss commonly used drugs that may induce bleeding or delay coagulation time.
2. Discuss commonly used hemostatic agents.
3. Describe the mechanisms of action of heparin, low molecular weight heparin, oral anticoagulants, antiplatelet agents, thrombolytic enzymes, alteplase, and tPA.
4. Identify commonly used drugs that may interact with heparin, oral anticoagulants, antiplatelet agents, thrombolytic enzymes, alteplase, and tPA.
5. Discuss the usual methods of administering heparin, low molecular weight heparin, and antiplatelet agents.
6. Describe the technique for subcutaneous (SC) administration of heparin and low molecular weight heparin.
7. Discuss safety measures used by nurses in providing care to clients receiving heparin, antiplatelet agents, or oral anticoagulants.
8. Apply the nursing process used in providing care for clients receiving heparin, antiplatelets, or oral anticoagulants.
9. Explain the general guidelines for safe intermittent administration of heparin using a saline lock.
10. Discuss the educational needs of clients receiving heparin, oral anticoagulants, or both.
11. Apply the nursing process for a client following intracoronary thrombolysis, using urokinase, streptokinase, alteplase, or tPA.
12. Successfully complete the games and activities in the online student StudyWARE.

Definitions

Supply the definitions for the following terms.

1. anticoagulant _____
2. heparin _____
3. hypoprothrombinemia _____
4. desmopressin acetate (DDAVP) _____
5. thrombus _____
6. hemostatic agents _____

Fill in the Blank

Write in the missing information.

1. The anticoagulant potency of heparin sodium injection is standardized by _____.
2. Overdoses of heparin can be treated with _____.
3. Some drugs/herbs that may decrease the effects of heparin include _____, _____, _____, _____, _____, _____, and _____.
4. The action of oral anticoagulants is not evident for at least _____ hours after the first dose has been administered.
5. _____ and _____ are the blood levels monitored for clients receiving oral anticoagulants.

6. Dosage of oral anticoagulants should be made to achieve and maintain a prothrombin time of _____ times the control value.

7. The effectiveness of heparin therapy is monitored by _____ times.

8. Heparin is not effective when administered _____.

9. The preferred routes for administration of heparin are _____ and _____.

10. _____ is an injectable antiplatelet drug used with aspirin and heparin to prevent coronary vessel occlusion in clients undergoing percutaneous transluminal coronary angioplasty or arthrectomy.

Multiple Choice

Circle the best answer for each of the following questions. There is only one answer to each question.

1. Alteplase recombinant is used to treat acute ischemic cerebrovascular accidents. It is most effective in decreasing residual effects of a stroke if given
   A. 24 hours after the stroke
   B. within the first 3 hours following the stroke
   C. for 8 hours following the stroke
   D. instead of heparin to treat this type of stroke

2. The nurse is obtaining a history from a client for whom heparin therapy is ordered. Which of the following drugs does the nurse identify as decreasing the effects of heparin?
   A. digitalis
   B. furosemide (Lasix)
   C. morphine sulfate
   D. ibuprofen

3. The nurse would anticipate use of heparin therapy for the treatment of a client with a diagnosis of
   A. dissecting aneurysm
   B. ulcerative colitis
   C. acute coronary syndrome
   D. threatened abortion

4. The nurse is working with a client who overused prescribed anticoagulants. Upon assessment, the nurse would expect to find which of the following?
   A. excessive hypoprothrombinemia
   B. angina
   C. low platelet counts
   D. increased red blood cell count

5. A client is receiving ticlopidine (Ticlid) to prevent recurrence of stroke. It is most important for the nurse to monitor the client for which adverse effect of the medication?
   A. hypertension
   B. renal failaure
   C. rash
   D. neutropenia

6. A client presents with a diagnosis of intermittent claudication. The nurse anticipates the client will receive treatment with which of the following medications?
   A. clopidogrel bisulfate (Plavix)
   B. ticlopidine (Ticlid)
   C. retaplase recombinant (Retavase)
   D. cilostazol (Pletal)

7. A client is undergoing a percutaneous transluminal coronary angioplasty. The nurse anticipates the client will be treated with aspirin, heparin, and which drug to prevent coronary vessel occlusion?
   A. tissue plasminogen activator (tPA)
   B. abciximab (ReoPro)
   C. desmopressin acetate (DDAVP)
   D. aprotinin (Trasylol)

8. A client is receiving Retaplase recombinant (Retavase) for the acute management of stroke. It is most important for the nurse to assess the client for the development of
   A. acute MI
   B. increased intracranial pressure
   C. intracranial hemorrhage
   D. thromboembolus

9. A client with hemophilia is undergoing surgery. The nurse anticipates use of which of the following medications during the surgical procedure?

    A. desmopressin acetate (DDAVP)
    B. aprotinin (Trasylol)
    C. thrombin
    D. aminocaproic acid (Amicar)

10. What laboratory values should the nurse monitor for clients receiving intravenous heparin therapy?

    A. prothrombin time (PT)
    B. international normalized ratio (INR)
    C. activated partial thromboplastin time (APTT)
    D. erythrocyte sedimentation rate

11. Which of the following instructions should the nurse include when teaching patients about oral anticoagulant therapy?

    A. monitor your capillary bleeding time
    B. wear a medical alert bracelet
    C. decrease your fluid intake
    D. take a vitamin K supplement daily if receiving heparin

12. A new nurse is administering subcutaneous heparin. Which action requires the supervising nurse to intervene? The new nurse

    A. uses the upper arm as the site to administer the heparin
    B. uses a 26-gauge needle
    C. uses a 5/8-inch needle
    D. uses the lateral abdominal wall as the site to administer the heparin

Multiple Response

Circle the best answer for each of the following questions. More than one answer is correct.

1. The nurse identifies which of the following statements about heparin therapy as true? Select all that apply.

    A. Heparin is not effective when administered orally.
    B. Intramuscular administration of heparin is not advised.
    C. The dosage of heparin should be expressed in USP units.
    D. Overdosage of heparin is treated with vitamin K.
    E. The half-life of heparin is 36 hours.
    F. Lovenox is a type of low molecular weight heparin.

2. Which of the following statements does the nurse include when teaching a client about oral anticoagulant therapy? Select all that apply.

    A. The oral anticoagulants inhibit blood clotting by interfering with the synthesis of vitamin C.
    B. The action of oral anticoagulants is evident in 90 minutes.
    C. Dosage of oral anticoagulants is determined by periodic determination of prothrombin time.
    D. The INR is monitored every 2–4 weeks for clients on oral anticoagulants.
    E. There are many drug interactions between oral anticoagulants and other drugs.
    F. Oral anticoagulants are primarily metabolized in the kidney.

3. When administering heparin subcutaneously, the nurse will do which of the following? Select all that apply.

    A. Use a U-100 insulin syringe.
    B. Select an injection site within 2 inches of the umbilicus.
    C. Apply ice in a plastic bag or rubber glove to the injection site before administration of the medication if the client experiences discomfort.
    D. Rub the desired site with antiseptic.
    E. Insert the needle at a 60-degree angle.
    F. Maintain pressure on the injection site for 10 seconds.

Critical Thinking Exercises

1. Compare and contrast the nursing responsibilities associated with care of the client receiving heparin and oral anticoagulant agents.

_____

_____

_____

_____

2. Create a care plan for a client receiving various antiplatelet agents.

_____

_____

_____

_____

3. Develop a poster to teach clients and families about the use of thrombolytic agents.

_____

_____

_____

_____

4. Develop a teaching plan for client self-administration of subcutaneous heparin.

_____

_____

_____

_____

5. Review nursing responsibilities associated with the care of a client after intracoronary thrombolysis using the protocol from a local health care facility.

_____

_____

_____

_____

CHAPTER 21 *Agents Used to Treat Anemias*

Objectives

After reading Chapter 21 of *Pharmacological Aspects of Nursing Care,* 8th edition, the student will be able to:

1. Discuss the manifestations of anemia.
2. Describe five groups at high risk for the development of iron deficiency anemia.
3. List three foods that are good sources of iron.
4. Discuss the advantages and disadvantages of oral, parenteral, and iron therapy.
5. Describe the treatment of iron overdose.
6. Discuss three causes of vitamin B_{12} deficiency.
7. List three foods that are good sources of vitamin B_{12}.
8. List three foods that are good sources of folic acid.
9. Differentiate among normocytic, microcytic, hypochromic, and megaloblastic red blood cells.
10. Discuss three drugs that can cause blood loss.
11. Apply the nursing process related to the administration of agents used in the treatment of anemias.
12. Successfully complete the games and activities in the online student StudyWARE.

Definitions

Supply the definitions for the following terms.

1. pernicious anemia _____
2. iron deficiency anemia _____
3. erythropoietin _____
4. cyanocobalamin _____
5. procrit _____

Fill in the Blank

Write in the missing information.

1. The mainstay treatment for iron deficiency anemia is _____.
2. Erythrocyte stimulant agents are contraindicated in the treatment of clients with _____.
3. When symptoms of anemia caused by B_{12} deficiency develop, they are usually characterized by _____, _____, and _____.
4. Supplementation with _____ during pregnancy has been shown to decrease the incidence of neural tube defects.
5. If too much iron accumulates in the body, a chelating agent _____ may be used to remove the excess iron through the kidney.

Multiple Choice

Circle the best answer for each of the following questions. There is only one answer to each question.

1. When assessing a client experiencing tissue hypoxia caused by anemia, the nurse anticipates the client will exhibit
   A. bradypnia
   B. bradycardia
   C. angina pectoris
   D. drowsiness

2. When working with clients with iron deficiency anemia, the nurse prepares to administer which of the following to stabilize the membrane of the red blood cell, protecting it from destruction?
   A. vitamin A
   B. vitamin D
   C. vitamin E
   D. vitamin K

3. The nurse identifies the most common cause of iron deficiency anemia as
   A. nutritional deficiency
   B. hematological disorders
   C. chemotherapy administration
   D. heredity

4. The nurse identifies the major site of gastrointestinal absorption of iron as the
   A. sigmoid colon
   B. proximal portion of the large intestine
   C. proximal portion of the small intestine
   D. distal portion of the stomach

5. Iron-deficient red blood cells are shaped
   A. macrocytic
   B. hypochromic and microcytic
   C. normocytic
   D. microcytic

6. The nurse identifies which of the following as the mainstay of treatment for clients with iron deficiency anemia?
   A. ferrous sulfate
   B. ferrous fumarate
   C. ferrous gluconate
   D. epogen

7. When instructing clients who are at the greatest risk of developing iron deficiency anemia about foods rich in iron, the nurse should include
   A. yellow vegetables
   B. citrus fruits
   C. dark green, leafy vegetables
   D. chicken breast meat

8. Clients with anemia caused by vitamin B_{12} deficiency are most likely to exhibit symptoms of
   A. diarrhea
   B. constipation
   C. bradycardia
   D. numbness and tingling of the extremities

9. The nurse identifies which of the following as a chelating agent used to remove excess iron from the body?
   A. deferoxamine mesylate
   B. hydroxocobalamin
   C. cyanocobalamin
   D. ferrous fumarate

10. Which of the following will the nurse include when teaching a client about deferoxamine mesylate therapy?
    A. pernicious anemia may result from treatment
    B. your urine may be colored red from the medication
    C. your skin may turn orange
    D. you may develop angina

Multiple Response

Circle the best answers for each of the following questions. More than one answer is correct.

1. When assessing a client with vitamin B_{12} deficiency, the nurse expects the client to exhibit which of the following? Select all that apply.
   A. tetany
   B. urticaria
   C. pitting edema
   D. sore tongue
   E. numbing and tingling of the arms
   F. numbing and tingling of the legs

2. Which of the following statements about folic acid deficiency does the nurse identify as being true? Select all that apply.
   A. Clients using methotrexate may need more folic acid.
   B. Clients receiving corticosteroids should not receive folic acid supplementation.
   C. Clients who are alcoholics may need folic acid supplementation.
   D. Pregnant women who take folic acid supplements have an increase in the incidence of children born with neural tube defects.
   E. Folic acid supplementation results in multiple severe adverse effects.
   F. Clients receiving phenytoin may need folic acid supplementation.

Critical Thinking Exercises

1. Discuss the types of anemia and describe their signs, symptoms, and treatment.

2. Develop a teaching plan for clients receiving folic acid supplementation.

3. Prepare a chart focusing on the nursing responsibilities in the administration of epogen and procrit. Focus on client safety.

4. Create a teaching plan for a client taking iron supplements, including nursing interventions. Specify techniques for promoting client safety.

5. Develop a plan of care for a client with vitamin B_{12} deficiency.

CHAPTER 22 *Vitamins, Minerals, and Other Nutritional Agents*

Objectives

After reading Chapter 22 of *Pharmacological Aspects of Nursing Care,* 8th edition, the student will be able to:

1. Discuss the roles of protein, fat, and carbohydrate in human nutrition.
2. Discuss the major vitamins and minerals required for health.
3. Identify common misconceptions about the purpose of and requirements for vitamins and minerals.
4. Discuss several common causes of hypokalemia, potassium, sodium, chloride, and other electrolyte imbalances.
5. Compare the fat-soluble and water-soluble vitamins and indicate the common circumstances in which a deficiency of each could occur.
6. Apply the nursing process associated with the administration of vitamin and mineral preparations.
7. Explain the function of the nurse in providing nutritional education.
8. Apply the nursing process for clients receiving total parenteral nutrition (TPN).
9. Successfully complete the games and activities in the online student StudyWARE.

Definitions

Supply the definitions for the following terms.

1. vitamins _____
2. minerals _____
3. fat-soluble vitamins _____
4. water-soluble vitamins _____
5. lipoproteins _____
6. proteins _____
7. carbohydrates _____
8. fats _____
9. hypernatremia _____
10. macronutrients _____

Fill in the Blank

Write in the missing information.

1. The micronutrients are the _____ and _____.
2. Vitamin _____ is necessary for the absorption of iron.
3. Less than _____ % of the daily caloric intake should come from saturated fats.
4. _____ is an essential factor for the normal biosynthesis of various blood clotting factors.
5. A deficiency of _____ causes a disorder known as beriberi.
6. An increase in the use of _____ in pregnant women has been found to decrease the incidence of neural tube anomalies.
7. The most serious manifestation of hypokalemia is the development of _____.
8. Calcium deficiency is manifested as _____ in the newborn infant.

Multiple Choice

Circle the best answer for each of the following questions. There is only one answer to each question.

1. Clients with a deficiency of which of the following minerals are most likely to experience tetany?

   A. calcium
   B. iron
   C. phosphorus
   D. magnesium

2. Which of the following vitamins is most likely to cause a greenish yellow fluorescence to the urine?

   A. thiamine
   B. riboflavin
   C. pyridoxine
   D. pantothenic acid

3. The nurse identifies which of the following as the most common cause of hyponatremia?

   A. hypertension
   B. peripheral edema
   C. severe diarrhea and vomiting
   D. polyuria

4. The nurse identifies which of the following as the most common cause of hypokalemia?

   A. nausea
   B. hyperaldosteronism
   C. hypernatremia
   D. respiratory alkalosis

5. The nurse identifies the two most serious complications of hypokalemia as cardiac arrhythmias and

   A. convulsions
   B. muscle cramps
   C. sensitization to digitalis-like drugs
   D. osteoporosis

6. The nurse anticipates administration of which drug for the treatment of acute hyperkalemia?

   A. calcium gluconate
   B. sodium bicarbonate
   C. sodium fluoride
   D. sodium polystyrene sulfonate

7. The nurse should monitor the client receiving calcium supplements in therapeutic doses over long periods of time for the development of

   A. hypocalcemia
   B. hyperalbuminemia
   C. hyperuricemia
   D. hypercalciuria

8. Which agent is sometimes included in iron supplement products to increase absorption of iron from the gastrointestinal tract?

   A. ascorbic acid
   B. niacin
   C. vitamin A
   D. essential amino acids

9. The nurse anticipates administration of which of the following agents for a client on renal dialysis who has developed hypermagnesia?

   A. calcium supplements
   B. aluminum
   C. sodium polystyrene sulfonate
   D. sorbitol

10. The nurse identifies which of the following as a trace element?

    A. sodium
    B. magnesium
    C. chloride
    D. copper

11. Which of the following is considered to be a routine dose of potassium added to a liter of intravenous fluid in a client who has had surgery?

    A. 20 mEq/L
    B. 30 mEq/L
    C. 40 mEq/L
    D. 50 mEq/L

12. When a central venous access device is used to deliver TPN, the client is most at risk for the development of

    A. hypoglycemia
    B. infection
    C. deficient fluid volume
    D. malnutrition

Multiple Response

Circle the best answers for each of the following questions. More than one answer is correct.

1. When administering potassium supplementation, the nurse will do which of the following? Select all that apply.
   A. Question an order for 100 mEq/L of potassium.
   B. Place a client on a cardiac monitor if the potassium supplement is more than 20mEq/L.
   C. Administer oral potassium supplements to a client on an empty stomach.
   D. Crush potassium tablets for oral administration to make them easier for the client to swallow.
   E. Administer intravenous potassium chloride that is diluted in D5W.
   F. Assess the client for cardiac arrhythmias.

2. The nurse identifies which of the following as interventions for clients experiencing hyponatremia? Select all that apply.
   A. restrict the intake of fluids
   B. administration of furosemide
   C. administration of 0.9% normal saline
   D. daily weight
   E. administration of D5W
   F. administration of sodium free fluids

Critical Thinking Exercises

1. Research the types of vitamins and minerals, comparing the recommended daily intakes with common intake practices.

   _____

   _____

   _____

   _____

2. Describe the effects of vitamins, minerals, carbohydrates, proteins, and fats, along with their contraindications.

   _____

   _____

   _____

   _____

3. Create a nutritional and weight loss plan for a client with renal failure and hypertension.

   _____

   _____

   _____

   _____

4. Compare treatment of clients with hyperkalemia and hypokalemia.

   _____

   _____

   _____

   _____

5. Develop a chart highlighting the treatment of clients with hyponatremia or hypernatremia.

_____

_____

_____

_____

CHAPTER 23 Agents Used to Treat Hyperacidity and Gastroesophageal Reflux Disease

Objectives

After reading Chapter 23 of *Pharmacological Aspects of Nursing Care,* 8th edition, the student will be able to:

1. Explain why some antacids cause constipation, and why others cause diarrhea.
2. Discuss three ways antacids may interact with other drugs.
3. Identify three prescription drugs that should not be administered with an antacid.
4. Differentiate among the actions of histamine H2 antagonists and proton pump inhibitors with antacids in the treatment of hyperacidity and gastroesophageal reflux disease (GERD).
5. Discuss adverse effects and drug or herbal interactions associated with proton pump inhibitors.
6. Discuss adverse effects and drug or herbal interactions associated with H2 antagonists.
7. Apply the nursing process related to caring for clients receiving agents used to treat hyperacidity and GERD.
8. Successfully complete the games and activities in the online student StudyWARE.

Definitions

Supply the definitions for the following terms.

1. hyperchlorhydria _____
2. *H. pylori* _____
3. misoprostol _____
4. sucralfate _____
5. metoclopramide _____

Fill in the Blank

Write in the missing information.

1. Simethicone is an antigas agent used in the management of clients with peptic ulcer disease.
2. Cimetidine is known to produce antiandrogenic effects and ___CNS___ effects.
3. Esomeprazole is a proton pump inhibitor that has been found to improve symptoms in up to 70% of clients with gastroesophageal reflux disease.
4. Misoprostol is a drug specifically indicated for the prevention of gastric ulcers produced by the use of nonsteroidal anti-inflammatory drugs (NSAIDs).
5. Dairy products that are lower in lactose include __yogurt__ and __hard cheese__

Multiple Choice

Circle the best answer for each of the following questions. There is only one answer to each question.

1. The nurse understands the use of antacids in the management of clients with peptic ulcer disease as their ability to

   A. heal gastric ulcers
   B. heal erosions of the esophagus
   C. treat the pain associated with peptic ulcer disease (PUD)
   D. reduce acid production by the stomach

2. The nurse identifies the most common adverse effect of magnesium oxide as

   A. diarrhea
   B. leukopenia
   C. hypertension
   D. hypocalcemia

3. When teaching a client prescribed antacids, which of the following does the nurse include?

   A. "Take the antacid with your other medications."
   B. "Taking the antacid as prescribed will heal the ulcer."
   C. "This medication with relieve pain associated with the ulcer."
   D. "Using this medication will prevent other ulcers from developing."

4. The nurse will teach a client diagnosed with peptic ulcer disease to avoid which of the following?

   A. acetaminophen
   B. antacids
   C. aspirin
   D. proton-pump inhibitors

5. The nurse identifies which of the following medications as being an ulcerogenic agent?

   A. acetaminophen
   B. allopurinol
   C. cyclobenzaprine
   D. indomethacin

6. The nurse will assess clients receiving aluminum hydroxide gel for the development of which electrolyte disturbance most likely to occur as a result of use of this agent?

   A. hyponatremia
   B. hypophosphatemia
   C. hypernatremia
   D. hyperkalemia

7. Which statement by a client receiving calcium carbonate indicates that more teaching is needed?

   A. "Use of this drug may increase acid in my stomach."
   B. "This drug can be used to prevent osteoporosis."
   C. "Use of this drug may cause gas bubbles to be released in my stomach."
   D. "Diarrhea most often occurs when using this drug."

8. Which of the following statements about proton pump inhibitors does the nurse identify as being true?

   A. These drugs suppress gastric acid secretion.
   B. Esomeprazole is used to treat *H. pylori*.
   C. Omeprazole is used to heal the esophagus.
   D. Lansoprazole is used for the treatment of children with peptic ulcer disease.

9. Which of the following agents does the nurse expect to be prescribed for the client receiving nonsteroidal anti-inflammatory agents to prevent gastric ulcer formation?

   A. esomeprazole
   B. misoprostol
   C. sucralfate
   D. metoclopramide

10. A client is prescribed metoclopramide. It is most important for the client to notify the health care provider if this client has a history of

    A. seizure disorder
    B. receiving chemotherapy
    C. gastroesophageal reflux disease
    D. gastroparesis

Multiple Response

Circle the best answers for each of the following questions. More than one answer is correct.

1. Which of the following will the nurse include when teaching the client about the use of sucralfate? Select all that apply.
   A. This drug is used to decrease the amount of acid your stomach makes.
   B. Sucralfate is usually used daily for 6 months before a benefit of the drug is evident.
   C. Take an antacid with sucralfate.
   D. Take the drug on an empty stomach.
   E. If you develop constipation, stop taking the drug.
   F. Nausea is a common adverse effect of use of this drug.

2. The nurse identifies which of the following conditions as a contraindication for the use of metoclopramide? Select all that apply.
   A. gastroparesis
   B. gastrointestinal perforation
   C. gastrointestinal obstruction
   D. gastrointestinal hemorrhage
   E. nausea
   F. vomiting

Critical Thinking Exercises

1. Visit a store that sells drugs used to treat hyperacidity and gastroesophageal reflux disease. How many varieties of drugs did you find? Share your results with the group.

   _____

   _____

   _____

   _____

2. Develop a teaching plan for a client with peptic ulcer disease focusing on pharmacologic treatment and client safety.

   _____

   _____

   _____

   _____

3. Develop a teaching plan for a client with pancreatic enzyme deficiency and lactase enzyme deficiency. Compare and contrast nursing interventions associated with administration of these agents.

   _____

   _____

   _____

   _____

CHAPTER 24 Antiemetics and Emetics

Objectives

After reading Chapter 24 of *Pharmacological Aspects of Nursing Care,* 8th edition, the student will be able to:

1. Discuss the common causes of nausea and vomiting.
2. Discuss the action of each of the classifications of agents in the treatment of nausea and vomiting.
3. Discuss when ipecac syrup is used in the emergency treatment of poisoning.
4. Apply the nursing process for clients receiving emetic and antiemetic agents.
5. Successfully complete the games and activities in the online student StudyWARE.

Definitions

Supply the definitions for the following terms.

1. 5-HT3 receptor antagonists _____
2. antiemetics _____
3. neuroleptic agents _____
4. prokinetic agents _____
5. promethazine HCl _____
6. ondansetron HCl _____

Fill in the Blank

Write in the missing information.

1. Anticholinergic side effects include _dry mouth_ , _urinary retention_ , and _blurred vision_ .
2. Some of the adverse effects of neuroleptic agents include _orthostatic hypotension_ , _sedation_ , and _tardative dyske_
3. The first 5-HT3 receptor antagonist developed was _ondansetron_
4. Extrapyramidal reactions occurring as a result of use of metoclopramide are treated with _diphenhydramine_
5. Clients prescribed meclizine should be instructed to take the medication _1 hour_ before departure.

Multiple Choice

Circle the best answer for each of the following questions. There is only one answer to each question.

1. The nurse recognizes the most common adverse effect associated with ondansetron HCl therapy as

   A. nausea
   B. diarrhea
   C. somnolence
   D. hypotension

2. A client is prescribed ondansetron HCl before initiation of chemotherapy. If the chemotherapy is prescribed to begin at 0800, when should the nurse administer the ondasetrom HCl?

   A. 0600
   B. 0730
   C. 0900
   D. 1200

3. Ondansetron is administered primarily for which of the following conditions?

   A. gastroesophageal reflux disease
   B. constipation
   C. peptic ulcer disease
   D. chemotherapy-induced nausea

4. A new nurse is preparing to administer prochlorperazine. The supervising nurse needs to intervene if the nurse attempts to administer the medication by which route?

   A. oral

   B. rectal

   C. intramuscularly

   D. subcutaneously

5. When administering anticholinergics for the tratment of nausea, the nurse identifies which of the following conditions as a contraindication for use of these agents?

   A. bradydysrhythmias

   B. acute renal failure

   C. peptic ulcer disease

   D. increased intraocular pressure

6. Chemotherapy-induced nausea and vomiting is most commonly treated with

   A. neuroleptics

   B. prokinetic agents

   C. 5-HT3 receptor antagonists

   D. antihistamines

7. The nurse identifies which of the following as an adverse effect from use of antihistamines?

   A. increased risk of urinary retention in client with benign prostatic hypertrophy

   B. increased urinary frequency resulting from overactive bladder

   C. worsening of diarrhea in client with Crohn's disease

   D. increased perspiration associated with elevated glucose levels

8. When a client is receiving droperidol, it is most important for the nurse to assess for which adverse effect?

   A. hypertension

   B. headache

   C. QT prolongation

   D. somnolence

9. Clients receiving scopolamine HCl patch should be instructed to remove the patch every

   A. 12 hours

   B. 24 hours

   C. 48 hours

   D. 72 hours

Multiple Response

Circle the best answers for each of the following questions. More than one answer is correct.

1. Which of the following drugs does the nurse identify as most effective in the treatment of nausea and vomiting associated with use of chemotherapy? Select all that apply.

   A. scopolamine

   B. diphenhydramine

   C. meclizine

   D. granisetron HCl

   E. palonosetron HCl

   F. ondansetron HCl

2. Which of the following will the nurse include when teaching a client about the use of antiemetic agents? Select all that apply.

   A. Avoid direct sunlight when taking promethazine HCl.

   B. Restrict fluids when taking diphenhydramine.

   C. Prochlorperazine may cause amenorrhea.

   D. Extrapyramidal reactions can occur when using metoclopramide.

   E. Clients taking perphenazine should rise slowly from sitting position.

   F. Ondansetron is primarily used for the treatment of postoperative nausea and vomiting from anesthesia.

Critical Thinking Exercises

1. Describe nursing responsibilities associated with each type of antiemetic focusing on client safety.

_____

_____

_____

_____

2. Prepare a chart describing use of antiemetic agents in the treatment of clients with nausea and vomiting associated with chemotherapeutic agents.

_____

_____

_____

_____

3. Talk with an oncology clinical specialist nurse about current and future treatment of chemotherapy-induced nausea and vomiting.

_____

_____

_____

_____

CHAPTER 25 *Laxatives and Antidiarrheals*

Objectives

After reading Chapter 25 of *Pharmacological Aspects of Nursing Care,* 8th edition, the student will be able to:

1. Describe five characteristics of an "ideal" laxative agent.
2. Explain the mechanism of action, common adverse effects, and drug interactions related to the use of the major laxative and antidiarrheal drugs.
3. Discuss the differences among the major categories of laxative agents.
4. Discuss the purpose for using stool softeners and bowel cleansing agents.
5. Discuss five possible causes of diarrhea and suggest therapeutic management of each.
6. Describe the procedure for the administration of a nonretention enema, including the modifications necessary because of the client's age.
7. Describe the procedure for the administration of a rectal suppository.
8. Apply the nursing process in caring for clients receiving laxatives and antidiarrheal agents.
9. Successfully complete the games and activities in the online student StudyWARE.

Definitions

Supply the definitions for the following terms.

1. stool softeners _____
2. bulk-forming laxatives _____
3. constipation _____
4. lactulose _____
5. lubricant laxatives _____
6. diarrhea _____
7. antidiarrheals _____
8. laxative dependence _____

Fill in the Blank

Write in the missing information.

1. The *stimulant laxatives* increase the motility of the gastrointestinal tract by chemical irritation of the intestinal mucosa or by a more selective action on specific nerves in the intestinal wall.
2. *hyperosmolar laxatives* exert their effect by drawing water through the intestinal wall by osmotic action and thereby increasing the fluidity of the stool and stimulating greater intestinal motility.
3. Biscodyl should not be administered within 1 hour of ingesting *milk*.
4. Lubricant laxatives are *oils* that act as lubricants to facilitate the passage of the fecal mass through the intestine.
5. The two classes of drugs used to treat diarrhea are *opium derivatives* and *anticholinergic agents*.

Multiple Choice

Circle the best answer for each of the following questions. There is only one answer to each question.

1. When working with clients receiving bulk forming laxatives, the nurse will
   A. assess for paralytic ileus as a common adverse effect when using these agents
   B. expect a response from use of the medication within 8 hours
   C. assess the client for indications of systemic absorption of the drug
   D. administer these agents with a large volume of fluid

2. When working with clients taking antidiarrheal medications containing opiates, it is most important for the nurse to monitor the client for the development of
   A. dependence   C. renal failure
   B. hypertension   D. seizures

3. Which of the following statements about stimulant laxatives does the nurse identify as being true?
   A. They act only on the small intestine.
   B. They tend to produce a watery, often diarrheal stool.
   C. They are not absorbed into the systemic circulation.
   D. Of all laxatives, they are least likely to cause laxative dependence.

4. Which of the following statements by a client taking polycarbophil indicates that more teaching is needed?
   A. "It is used to treat diarrhea."
   B. "It works by decreasing movement of the intestine."
   C. "It is used to treat constipation."
   D. "It will restore a normal moisture level to the colon."

5. Nurses should teach clients to use caution when driving or operating heavy equipment when taking which of the following medications?
   A. senna   C. psyllium
   B. diphenoxylate HCl   D. docusate sodium

6. The nurse will teach clients taking which of the following agents that their stool may be discolored?
   A. psyllium   C. cascara sagrada
   B. biscodyl   D. senna

7. When administering saline laxatives, it is most important for the nurse to assess the client for a history of
   A. asthma C. diabetes mellitus
   B. renal insufficiency D. scleroderma

8. A laxative is ordered for a client with chronic renal failure. Which medication order will the nurse question?
   A. sodium phosphate   C. casara sagrada
   B. senna   D. biscodyl

9. Which statement by a client taking bisacodyl indicates that more teaching is needed?
   A. "I will take the tablet whole."
   B. "I will take the tablet with milk to prevent stomach problems."
   C. "I will avoid taking milk with this medication."
   D. "I may experience diarrhea from taking this drug."

10. It is most important for the nurse to teach clients taking bulk-forming laxatives to
    A. always administer them via enema
    B. expect to experience frequent diarrhea
    C. prepare for effects of the medication to occur within 6 hours
    D. take the medication with a large volume of fluid

Multiple Response

Circle the best answers for each of the following questions. More than one answer is correct.

1. Which of the following statements about *Lactobacillus acidophilus* does the nurse identify as being true? Select all that apply.
   A. It is normally found in the gastrointestinal tract.
   B. It is used for the treatment of diarrhea associated with antibiotic therapy.
   C. It should be stored in the refrigerator.
   D. It must not be administered with yogurt.
   E. Use of milk is contraindicated with these agents.

2. Which of the statements regarding the treatment of diarrhea does the nurse identify as true? Select all that apply.
   A. Diarrhea is a symptom of an underlying disorder.
   B. Diarrhea can be a life-threatening condition.
   C. Drug therapy is aimed at increasing motility of the gastrointestinal tract.
   D. Adsorbents are the most commonly used antidiarrheal agents.
   E. Anticholinergic agents can be used to treat diarrhea.
   F. Loperamide HCl is the treatment of choice for children under the age of 2 who have diarrhea.

Critical Thinking Exercises

1. Discuss nursing responsibilities associated with major types of stimulant, bulk-forming, lubricant, and hyperosmotic laxatives, as well as stool softeners. Include their mechanisms of action, and provide two examples of each.

   _____

   _____

   _____

   _____

2. Create a teaching plan for a client taking antidiarrheal agents.

   _____

   _____

   _____

   _____

3. Compare and contrast nursing responsibilities associated with children and adults prescribed laxatives and antidiarrheals.

   _____

   _____

   _____

   _____

CHAPTER 26 *Central Nervous System Sedatives and Hypnotics*

Objectives

After reading Chapter 26 of *Pharmacological Aspects of Nursing Care,* 8th edition, the student will be able to:

1. Explain the difference between a drug used as a sedative and one used as a hypnotic.
2. Discuss four classes of drugs that may interact with barbiturate sedative-hypnotics.
3. Discuss the therapeutic effects and adverse effects of the major barbiturate, benzodiazepene, and nonbarbiturate sedative-hypnotics.
4. Explain general supportive nursing interventions used in the treatment of sleep pattern disturbances.
5. Apply the nursing process related to the administration of each of the barbiturate, benzodiazepene, and nonbarbiturate sedative-hypnotic agents.
6. Successfully complete the games and activities in the online student StudyWARE.

Definitions

Supply the definitions for the following terms.

1. sedatives _____
2. benzodiazepines _____
3. barbiturates _____
4. hypnotics _____
5. ethanol _____

Fill in the Blank

Write in the missing information.

1. *Benzodiazepines* are often used as hypnotic agents for clients who need therapy for longer than 1–2 weeks.
2. *Flumazenil* is the drug used to reverse midazolam.
3. Some herbs used to promote sleep include *kava rhizome* and *Valerian root*
4. Clients with *asthma* and *glaucoma* should be cautioned not to use nonprescription sleep aids.
5. Phenobarbitol exerts a fairly selective action on the motor cortex and produces an *anticonvulsant* action as well.

Multiple Choice

Circle the best answer for each of the following questions. There is only one answer to each question.

1. The nurse identifies which of the following drugs as most likely to cause tissue extravasation?
   A. secobarbitol sodium
   B. butabarbital sodium
   C. pentobarbitol sodium
   D. estazolam

2. The nurse identifies the most common use of benzodiazepines as management of
   A. insomnia
   B. hysteria
   C. anxiety
   D. psychosis

3. A new nurse is preparing to administer pentobarbitol sodium to a client. Which action by the nurse requires the supervising nurse to intervene? The new nurse

   A. discards a parenteral solution if a precipitate is present
   B. assesses the IV line for patency
   C. prepares to administer the drug in the gluteus maximus
   D. prepares to administer pentobarbitol sodium in the same syringe as meperidine HCl

4. The nurse identifies the most common indication for use of eszopiclone as *Lunesta*

   A. pre-procedural sedation
   B. treatment for sleep disorders
   C. adjunct treatment for epilepsy
   D. treatment of anxiety disorders

5. The nurse identifies which of the following drugs as most likely to be considered a non-habit-forming agent?

   A. chloral hydrate
   B. zaleplon
   C. zolpidem tartrate
   D. trazodone

6. When administering chloral hydrate to a client, the nurse is aware that this drug is most likely to affect dosage requirements of which of the following drugs?

   A. insulin
   B. digoxin
   C. anticoagulants
   D. beta blockers

7. When teaching clients about the use of nonprescription sleep aids, it is most important for the nurse to inform clients with a history of which condition to notify their health care provider before taking these medications?

   A. cataracts
   B. rheumatoid arthritis
   C. psoriasis
   D. asthma

8. When working with clients receiving which of the following medications does the nurse identify that rapid discontinuation of these mediations may cause coma, convulsions, or death?

   A. barbiturates
   B. benzodiazepines
   C. anxiolytics
   D. sleep aids

9. A client is scheduled for a procedure requiring conscious sedation. The nurse anticipates administration of which drug?

   A. temazepam
   B. midazolam
   C. secobarbital sodium
   D. estazolam

Multiple Response

Circle the best answers for each of the following questions. More than one answer is correct.

1. When teaching a client with a sleep disorder, which of the following will the nurse include? Select all that apply.

   A. Determine if the client is taking antiparkinson drugs as they may interfere with sleep.
   B. Determine if the client is taking calcium-channel blocking drugs as they may interfere with sleep.
   C. Tell client to keep medication for sleep at bedside so it is convenient for use.
   D. Discussing starting a routine for going to bed.
   E. Encourage exercise during the day as it has been found to enhance sleep.
   F. Avoid use of any type of pain relief drug with medication to aid in sleep.

2. Which of the following does the nurse associate with barbiturate toxicity? Select all that apply.

   A. confusion
   B. excitement
   C. heavy sleep
   D. dry skin
   E. hypertension
   F. cyanosis

Critical Thinking Exercises

1. List major types of barbiturates, sedatives, and hypnotic medications. Discuss their mechanisms of action, and provide two examples of each. Include nursing responsibilities associated with administration of these medications.

   _____

   _____

   _____

   _____

2. List major types of benzodiazepines, and describe the nursing responsibilities associated with their use in client care.

   _____

   _____

   _____

   _____

3. Create a care plan for a client taking sedatives and hypnotics, including interventions and ways to maintain client safety.

   _____

   _____

   _____

   _____

CHAPTER 27 *Anxiolytics and Other Agents Used to Treat Psychiatric Health Alterations*

Objectives

After reading Chapter 27 of *Pharmacological Aspects of Nursing Care,* 8th edition, the student will be able to:

1. Describe the major classes of psychotropic agents and give an example of an agent in each class.
2. Discuss the mechanism of action of the major classes of psychotropic agents.
3. Describe the major therapeutic and adverse effects associated with the use of each class of psychotropic agents.
4. Discuss the drug interactions associated with psychotropic agents.
5. Explain the observations the nurse should make when a client is receiving a psychotropic agent to assess its effectiveness or presence of adverse effects.
6. Discuss the antipsychotic agents that may be administered on a once-daily schedule and discuss the advantage of this regimen.
7. Apply the nursing process related to providing care for clients receiving each of the classes of agents used in the treatment of psychiatric disorders.
8. Successfully complete the games and activities in the online student StudyWARE.

Definitions

Supply the definitions for the following terms.

1. psychotropic drugs _____
2. biogenic amine hypothesis _____
3. neuroleptics _____
4. affective disorders _____
5. tardive dyskinesia _____
6. anxiolytics _____
7. monoamine oxidase inhibitors _____
8. serotonin _____

Fill in the Blank

Write in the missing information.

1. The four groups of drugs currently used in the United States for the treatment of anxiety are *barbiturates carbamates*, *antihistamines*, and *benzodiazepines*
2. _Doxepin_ is a miscellaneous anxiolytic with a rapid onset of action.
3. The first-line agents used for the treatment of depression and anxiety are the _SSRI's_.
4. When antidepressant therapy is begun, therapeutic effects may not be evident until _2-3 weeks_ of therapy have elapsed.
5. The first antipsychotic agent to be introduced was _thorazine_.
6. _Akathisia_ is the subjective feeling of restlessness resulting in an inability to sit still.
7. _____ is an extrapyramidal symptom that usually appears after a client has been receiving antipsychotic drug therapy for more than 2 years.
8. _Antipsychotic_ drugs are primarily used in the treatment of schizophrenia.

Multiple Choice

Circle the best answer for each of the following questions. There is only one answer to each question.

1. The nurse identifies which of the following statements about benzodiazepines as being true?
   A. Benzodiazepines suppress REM sleep.
   B. These agents do not readily cause the development of tolerance.
   C. Benzodiazepines cause excessive drowsiness at therapeutic doses.
   D. These agents do not interfere with the metabolism of other drugs.

2. A client taking antipsychotic medications presents with fever, muscle rigidity, altered consciousness, and alterations in vital signs. The nurse prepares to provide treatment for
   A. autonomic dysreflexia
   B. extrapyramidal symptoms
   C. neuroleptic malignant syndrome
   D. malignant hypertension

3. When working with a client receiving buspirone, the nurse will
   A. administer the drug with monoamine oxidase inhibitors
   B. administer the buspirone as needed
   C. use this drug for management of acute anxiety
   D. teach the client that optimal results of the drug will not be seen for 3–4 weeks

4. A client has received a toxic dose of a benzodiazepine. The nurse anticipates the administration of which of the following to reverse the central nervous system depressant effects?
   A. atropine
   B. narcan
   C. glucagon
   D. flumazenil

5. A client with narrow-angle glaucoma is ordered to receive an oral anxiolytic agent. The nurse should question administration of which of the following drugs?
   A. diazepam
   B. alprazolam
   C. lorazepam
   D. oxazepam

6. Clients receiving monoamine oxidase inhibitors should be taught to avoid foods that are high in
   A. protein
   B. tyramine
   C. fat
   D. riboflavin

7. Which statement by a client taking monoamine oxidase inhibitors indicates that teaching has been effective?
   A. "I will avoid red wine."
   B. "I will take the medication with aged cheese."
   C. "I will take the medication only when I don't feel well."
   D. "Pickled herring is a good snack for me to have."

8. Which statement by a client taking antipsychotic agents indicates that more teaching is needed?
   A. "I will get up slowly from a seated position."
   B. "I will not drive after taking this medication."
   C. "I can expect this drug to cause me to have diarrhea."
   D. "I will use hard candy to help with the dryness in my mouth."

Multiple Response

Circle the best answers to each of the following questions. More than one answer is correct.

1. A client has abruptly stopped taking an anxiolytic medication. Upon assessment of the client, the nurse expects to find which of the following? Select all that apply
   A. insomnia
   B. weakness
   C. anxiety
   D. irritability
   E. flaccid muscles
   F. rash

2. Which statements by a client taking monoamine oxidase inhibitors indicate that teaching has been effective? Select all that apply.
   A. "I will avoid hard cheese."
   B. "If I have a cold, I will call my primary care provider before taking any cold remedy."
   C. "I will call my primary care provider if I experience a headache."
   D. "I can expect this medication to cause my heart to beat irregularly."
   E. "I will have my blood pressure monitored regularly."
   F. "Avocados are a good snack for me to have."

Critical Thinking Exercises

1. Develop a chart of anxiolytic agents. Describe their mechanism of action and the nursing responsibilities associated with each type of agent.

   _____

   _____

   _____

   _____

2. Develop a teaching plan for a client receiving monoamine oxidase inhibitors focusing on client safety.

   _____

   _____

   _____

   _____

3. Develop a chart describing action and nursing responsibilities associated with the treatment of clients with depression.

   _____

   _____

   _____

   _____

4. Develop a teaching plan for a client receiving antispychotic drugs and his or her caregivers focusing on medication safety.

   _____

   _____

   _____

   _____

CHAPTER 28 *CNS Stimulants, Agents Used to Treat Attention-Deficit Hyperactivity Disorder and Alzheimer's Disease*

Objectives

After reading Chapter 28 of *Pharmacological Aspects of Nursing Care*, 8th edition, the student will be able to:

1. Discuss three indications for the use of central nervous system (CNS) stimulants.
2. Discuss three adverse effects associated with the use of anorectic drugs.
3. Describe three manifestations of attention-deficit hyperactivity disorder (ADHD).
4. Discuss the agents used as CNS stimulants.
5. Discuss the agents used to treat ADHD.
6. Discuss the agents used to treat the manifestations of Alzheimer's disease.
7. Explain specific nursing interventions related to the administration of agents used to treat ADHD.
8. Explain specific nursing interventions related to the administration of agents used to treat the symptoms of Alzheimer's disease.
9. Apply the nursing process related to the use of CNS stimulants, agents used to treat ADHD, and agents used to treat the symptoms of Alzheimer's disease.
10. Successfully complete the games and activities in the online student StudyWARE.

Definitions

Supply the definitions for the following terms.

1. tacrine HCl _____
2. attention-deficit hyperactivity disorder _____
3. Alzheimer's disease _____
4. analeptics _____
5. anorectic agents _____
6. memantine _____
7. doxapram HCl _____
8. narcolepsy _____

Fill in the Blank

Write in the missing information.

1. Microscopic changes with Alzheimer's disease include _neuro tangles_ and _senile plaques_
2. _Caffine_ is the most commonly used central nervous stimulant in nonprescription products.
3. The three principal characteristics of attention-deficit hyperactivity disorder are _attention_, _impulsivity_, and _hyperactivity_
4. _Caffine_ is sometimes used as a treatment for apnea in preterm neonates.
5. Clients with cholinergic crisis due to overdose of donepezil HCL are treated with _atropine_

Multiple Choice

Circle the best answer for each of the following questions. There is only one answer to each question.

1. The nurse must assess clients receiving which of the following drugs for the development of psychologic dependence, multiple drug interactions, and increased seizures in clients with a history of seizure disorder?

   A. diethylpropion HCl
   B. doxapram HCl
   C. methylphenidate HCl *Ritalin*
   D. benphetamine HCl

2. Which statement by a caregiver of a client with Alzheimer's disease indicates that more teaching is needed?

   A. "These medications will help my loved one return to normal."
   B. "My loved one will have a loss of memory."
   C. " Clients with Alzheimer's disease usually die from sepsis, aspiration, pneumonia, or another concurrent chronic illness."
   D. "People with Alzheimer's disease have physical changes in their brains."

3. The nurse will instruct the client to take their daily dose of amphetamine

   A. upon awakening
   B. at lunch
   C. with dinner
   D. at bed time

4. The nurse identifies which of the following statements about anorexiants as true?

   A. These agents are sympathomimetic agents.
   B. They increase appetite.
   C. No tolerance develops to these drugs.
   D. Bradycardia is a common adverse effect of these drugs.

5. Which of the following drugs used in the management of Alzheimer's disease works by increasing the levels of N-methyl-D-aspartate?

   A. donepezil
   B. rivastigmine
   C. memantine
   D. tacrine HCl

6. Before administering tacrine HCl to a client, it is most important for the nurse to assess the client for a history of

   A. chronic obstructive pulmonary disease
   B. liver disease
   C. kidney disease
   D. diabetes mellitus

7. Which statement by the caregiver of a client receiving donepezil for the treatment of Alzheimer's disease indicates teaching has been effective?

   A. "I will give this medication to my loved one on an empty stomach."
   B. "I will call the health care provider if my loved one develops nausea."
   C. "Agitation has been seen during the initial weeks of treatment, but it usually subsides."
   D. "I can expect my loved one to recover from Alzheimer's disease after taking this medication for 1 month."

8. The nurse identifies which of the following as an effect of rivastigmine in the treatment of Alzheimer's disease?

   A. increases agitation
   B. slow progression of the disease
   C. temporarily slows cognitive decline
   D. returns functioning to normal

9. The nurse identifies which agent used in the treatment of Alzheimer's disease as having a high incidence of adverse effects?

   A. donepezil
   B. rivastigmine
   C. galantamine HBr
   D. tacrine

10. When a client is taking benzphetamine HCl, it is most important for the nurse to assess the client for a history of

    A. hypertension
    B. asthma
    C. diabetes mellitus
    D. renal function

Multiple Response

Circle the best answers for each of the following questions. More than one answer is correct.

1. The nurse should teach clients receiving anorexiants to monitor medications for which of the following side effects? Select all that apply.
   A. insomnia
   B. bradycardia
   C. nervousness
   D. rash
   E. dizziness
   F. fatigue

2. Which of the following will the nurse include when teaching the client proper use of rivastigmine patch? Select all that apply.
   A. Keep the patch on for 48 hours.
   B. Remove the old patch before applying the new patch.
   C. Place the patch on your anterior chest.
   D. Place the patch on your upper back.
   E. Rotate the patch between four spots on your body using the same spot every 4 days.
   F. Remove the patch and replace it every 24 hours.

Critical Thinking Exercises

1. Develop a plan of care for a client taking anorexiants focusing on client safety.

2. Develop a plan of care for a caregiver of a child with ADHD. How will this plan differ when the child is in school and when the child is away from school?

3. Research pharmacologic management of the client with Alzheimer's disease. Develop a teaching program for nurses caring for clients with Alzheimer's disease focusing on medication therapy, and develop a teaching plan for caregivers of clients with Alzheimer's disease.

CHAPTER 29 *Agents Used to Treat Musculoskeletal Health Alterations*

Objectives

After reading Chapter 29 of *Pharmacological Aspects of Nursing Care,* 8th edition, the student will be able to:

1. Describe three uses for neuromuscular blocking agents.
2. Compare the mechanism of action of competitive and depolarizing neuromuscular blocking agents.
3. Discuss three drugs that may intensify the action of neuromuscular blocking agents.
4. Discuss the therapeutic effects, adverse effects, drug interactions, and routes of administration of the major neuromuscular blocking agents and centrally acting skeletal muscle relaxants.
5. Discuss the therapeutic effects, adverse effects, drug interactions, and routes of administration of agents used to treat osteoporosis.
6. Apply the nursing process related to administration of the major neuromuscular blocking and centrally acting skeletal muscle relaxants and stimulants.
7. Apply the nursing process in caring for clients being treated for osteoporosis.
8. Successfully complete the games and activities in the online student StudyWARE.

Definitions

Supply the definitions for the following terms.

1. neuromuscular blockade _____
2. centrally acting skeletal muscle relaxants _____
3. AChR antibody test _____
4. cholinergic crisis _____
5. ambenonium Cl _____

Fill in the Blank

Write in the missing information.

1. Antidotal drugs for neuromuscular blocking agents include _____ and _____.
2. _____ is a direct-acting skeletal muscle relaxant that does not interfere with neuromuscular transmission of the electrical excitability of muscle; it does appear to inhibit the release of calcium from the muscle.
3. _____ is a neuromuscular disease that results from damage to acetylcholine receptors at the neuromuscular junction caused by an autoimmune reaction.
4. _____ is one of the newest dopamine receptor agonists designated specifically for the treatment of restless legs syndrome.
5. _____ is an anticholinesterase muscle stimulant that must be taken at exactly the prescribed time to be effective.

Multiple Choice

Circle the best answer for each of the following questions. There is only one answer to each question.

1. Which of the following neuromuscular blocking agents does the nurse identify as most effective in the treatment of older clients?

   A. doxacurium chloride
   B. pancuronium bromide
   C. cisatracurium
   D. atracurium besylate

2. The nurse will teach clients taking which of the following centrally acting skeletal muscle relaxants that the medication may turn their urine an orange or purple-red color?

   A. baclofen
   B. carisoprodol
   C. chlorzoxazone
   D. cyclobenzaprine HCl

3. The nurse identifies which of the following neuromuscular blocking agents as most likely to cause malignant hyperthermia?

   A. mivacurium chloride
   B. pancuronium bromide
   C. rocuronium bromide
   D. succinylcholine chloride

4. The nurse identifies baclofen as most often used for the treatment of clients with

   A. spinal cord injuries
   B. tetanus
   C. muscle atonia
   D. muscle fatigue

5. The nurse identifies which of the following drugs as safe to administer to a client who is also receiving a neuromuscular blocker?

   A. acetaminophen
   B. aminoglycoside
   C. tetracycline
   D. cortisol

6. The supervising nurse needs to intervene if the new nurse prepares to administer a neuromuscular blocking agent for management of a client with

   A. mechanical ventilation
   B. electroconvulsive therapy
   C. myasthenia gravis
   D. head injury

7. Which of the following statements about the diagnosis of myasthenia gravis does the nurse identify as being true?

   A. Endrophonium is administered intravenously to diagnose myasthenia gravis.
   B. The AChR antibody test is negative in the majority of clients with myasthenia gravis.
   C. Epinephrine should be available to counteract adverse reactions to the medication used to diagnose myasthenia gravis.
   D. Pediatric clients cannot have myasthenia gravis so they should not be tested for it.

8. The nurse identifies which of the following statements about restless legs syndrome (RLS) as true?

   A. Use of caffeine decreases RLS symptoms.
   B. This syndrome is found only in clients who have diabetes mellitus.
   C. Ropinirole HCl has been found to be an effective treatment for RLS.
   D. Tricyclic antidepressants are used to treat RLS.

9. The nurse should teach the client with myasthenia gravis to take his or her medication

   A. at breakfast
   B. at lunch time
   C. with supper
   D. at bedtime

10. A client has cholinergic crisis. The nurse anticipates administration of

    A. pyridostigmine bromide
    B. epinephrine
    C. edrophonium chloride
    D. atropine

Multiple Response

Circle the best answers for each of the following questions. More than one answer is correct.

1. The nurse expects to find which of the following when assessing a client with myasthenic crisis? Select all that apply.

   A. muscle weakness
   B. dyspnea
   C. dysphagia
   D. bradycardia
   E. miosis
   F. intestinal cramping

2. Which of the following statements about dantrolene does the nurse identify as true? Select all that apply.

   A. Dantrolene inhibits the release of potassium from the muscle.
   B. It can be used for the treatment of malignant hyperthermia.
   C. It is used for the treatment of skeletal muscle spasms.
   D. Dantrolene can cause overt hepatitis.
   E. Clients taking this medication should avoid direct sunlight.
   F. Dantrolene interferes with neuromuscular transmission.

Critical Thinking Exercises

1. Compare and contrast use of neuromuscular blocking agents for care of clients in the operating room and in the intensive care unit.

   _____

   _____

   _____

   _____

2. Discuss nursing responsibilities associated with administration and management of the client receiving neuromuscular blocking agents.

   _____

   _____

   _____

   _____

3. Create a care plan for a client with myasthenia gravis focusing on medication management and client safety.

   _____

   _____

   _____

   _____

CHAPTER 30 *Agents Used to Treat Parkinson's Disease*

Objectives

After reading Chapter 30 of *Pharmacological Aspects of Nursing Care*, 8th edition, the student will be able to:

1. Explain the mechanism by which levodopa acts to treat the symptoms of Parkinson's disease.
2. Discuss the actions, drug interactions, and adverse effects of drugs when used in the treatment of Parkinson's disease.
3. Apply the nursing process related to the administration and use of the major antiparkinson agents.
4. Successfully complete the games and activities in the online student StudyWARE.

Definitions

Supply the definitions for the following terms.

1. carbidopa _____
2. amantadine _____
3. apromorphine _____
4. benztropine mesylate _____
5. levodopa _____

Fill in the Blank

Write in the missing information.

1. Parkinson's disease is a neurologic disorder characterized by _____, _____, and _____.
2. Experimental evidence has revealed that clients with PD have an excessive amount of _____ and a deficiency of _____.
3. All forms of treatment for PD are _____, not curative.
4. Levodopa therapy has been found to reactivate _____ in clients who have a history of this disease.
5. Clients receiving levodopa therapy should be instructed to avoid foods high in _____ and _____.

Multiple Choice

Circle the best answer for each of the following questions. There is only one answer to each question.

1. A client is experiencing a parkinsonism crisis from undermedication. The nurse anticipates administration of which of the following?
   A. amantadine HCl
   B. benztropine mesylate
   C. apomorphine
   D. carbidopa

2. The nurse will teach clients taking which drug for the treatment of Parkinson's disease that their urine may turn dark?
   A. entacapone
   B. levodopa
   C. selegiline HCl
   D. benztropine mesylate

3. The nurse identifies which of the following medications as most likely to effect a client's liver function?
   A. selegiline HCl
   B. bromocriptine mesylate
   C. levodopa
   D. tolcapone

4. A client has been prescribed levodopa therapy for the treatment of Parkinson's disease. It is most important for the nurse to assess the client for a history of
   A. hypertension
   B. systemic lupus erythmatosis
   C. diabestes mellitus
   D. malignant melanoma

5. The nurse teaches the client prescribed benztropine mesylate to take the once daily dose at what time of day?
   A. early morning
   B. midday
   C. bedtime
   D. noon

6. The nurse should monitor the client taking which of the following drugs for the treatment of Parkinson's disease for the possible adverse effect of purple mottling to the skin?
   A. levodopa
   B. selegiline HCl
   C. amantadine HCl
   D. trihexyphenidyl HCl

7. When performing a physical assessment on a client with Parkinson's disease, the nurse is most likely to find which of the following?
   A. atonia, paresthesia, skin rash
   B. rigidity, muscle tremors, bradycardia
   C. lack of coordination, muscle tremors, rigidity
   D. weak muscles, inability to maintain posture, hypertension

8. A client has been prescribed an anticholinergic medication for the treatment of Parkinson's disease. It is most important for the nurse to assess the client for a history of
   A. cataracts
   B. narrow-angle glaucoma
   C. seizure disorder
   D. pyelonephritis

9. Which of the following medications used to treat Parkinson's disease does the nurse identify as most likely to cause the client to experience abnormal movements?
   A. bromocriptine mesylate
   B. trihexphenidyl HCl
   C. entacapone
   D. selegiline HCl

10. The nurse should teach a client receiving levodopa therapy for the treatment of Parkinson's disease that meals high in what component should be avoided when taking the drug?
    A. fat
    B. carbohydrates
    C. protein
    D. fiber

Multiple Response

Circle the best answers for each of the following questions. More than one answer is correct.

1. Which of the following statements by a client receiving levodopa therapy indicate that teaching has been effective? Select all that apply.
   A. I will take the medication with egg whites.
   B. I will take the medication with fruit.
   C. I will take this medication with a fortified cereal.
   D. If my urine turns dark, I will stop taking the medication.
   E. I will get up slowly from a chair.
   F. I will contact the health care provider if I feel depressed.

2. Which of the following statements about entacapone therapy does the nurse identify as true? Select all that apply.
   A. This medication causes the client's urine to turn brown.
   B. An adverse effect of this medication is purple mottling of the skin.
   C. This medication must be administered subcutaneously.
   D. This medication is contraindicated if the client is receiving monoamine oxidase inhibitors (MAOs).
   E. It is important to monitor liver function tests for clients taking this medication.
   F. The client should be assessed for the development of extrapyramidal symptoms.

Critical Thinking Exercises

1. Compare and contrast nursing responsibilities associated with clients receiving various drugs used to treat Parkinson's disease.

_____

_____

_____

_____

2. Create a teaching plan for a client and caregiver of a client receiving drugs to treat Parkinson's disease focusing on client safety.

_____

_____

_____

_____

3. Consult a dietician at a local health care facility and investigate dietary needs of a client with Parkinson's disease.

_____

_____

_____

_____

CHAPTER 31 Agents Used to Treat Seizures/Epilepsy

Objectives

After reading Chapter 31 of *Pharmacological Aspects of Nursing Care,* 8th edition, the student will be able to:

1. Discuss the common manifestations of seizure disorders.
2. Distinguish between generalized and partial focal seizures.
3. Discuss five possible causes of seizure disorders.
4. Distinguish infantile spasms from other types of seizure activity.
5. Discuss the most commonly used anticonvulsants and indicate their major adverse effects.
6. Explain the important aspects of a client education program for a person just diagnosed as having a seizure disorder and started on anticonvulsants.
7. Discuss factors to be assessed in monitoring the effectiveness of anticonvulsant drug therapy.
8. Discuss three factors that can decrease the seizure threshold, thereby increasing the likelihood of seizures.
9. Discuss techniques of oral care that may decrease gum problems due to phenytoin (Dilantin) therapy.
10. Recognize the major classes of drugs that may interact with anticonvulsants.
11. Apply the nursing process for clients taking anticonvulsants.
12. Explain special nursing needs of clients receiving treatment for status epilepticus.
13. Successfully complete the games and activities in the online student StudyWARE.

Definitions

Supply the definitions for the following terms.

1. felbamate _____
2. acetazolamide _____
3. carbamazepine _____
4. absence seizure _____
5. generalized tonic-clonic seizure _____
6. diazepam _____
7. infantile seizures _____
8. status epilepticus _____
9. intractable seizures _____
10. AED _____

Fill in the Blank

Write in the missing information.

1. The most common adverse effects of phenytoin are experienced in the _____.
2. Because of the difficulty of starting an intravenous infusion during seizure activity, _____ may be given rectally during status epilepticus.
3. The nurse should carefully monitor clients on carbamazepine therapy for the deficiency of the electrolyte _____.
4. Zonisamide therapy has been associated with fatal reactions when it is administered with _____.
5. The nurse should avoid administration of diazepam via the _____ route.

Multiple Choice

Circle the best answer for each of the following questions. There is only one answer to each question.

1. The nurse identifies which of the following statements about seizure disorders as being true?

   A. Most clients with seizure disorders first exhibit symptoms after age 25.
   B. Generally, seizures that begin after the age of 20 are related to electrolyte imbalances.
   C. Seizures that begin after age 20 are usually associated with a primary lesion of the central nervous system.
   D. Clients with seizure disorder always have an associated impairment of the mental abilities.

2. The nurse identifies which of the following as the best definition of epilepsy?

   A. many types of recurrent seizures characterized by excessive electrical discharge of nerves in the cerebral cortex
   B. a series of continuous seizures
   C. a cognitive impairment resulting from abnormal electrical activity
   D. a series of electrical impulses stimulating more than one area of the brain at a time

3. The nurse correctly describes a focal lesion as

   A. the client focuses on the seizure
   B. the client loses consciousness
   C. uncontrolled electrical discharges that occur in a localized area of the central nervous system
   D. the seizures begin in a specific area

4. The nurse identifies the most common adverse effect of long-term therapy with phenytoin as

   A. leukocytopenia
   B. gingival hyperplasia
   C. anemia
   D. elevated erythrocyte sedimentation rate

5. When administering phenytoin via the intravenous route, the nurse will use which of the following solutions?

   A. dextrose 5% in water (D5W)
   B. 0.9% normal sterile saline (NSS)
   C. Lactated Ringer's
   D. 0.45% NSS

6. The nurse identifies which of the following drugs used in the management of clients with seizure disorders as most likely to cause aplastic anemia?

   A. valproic acid
   B. fosphenytoin sodium
   C. phenytoin
   D. carbamazepine

7. A client is receiving clonazepam therapy for the management of seizure disorder. It is most important for the nurse to assess the client for a history of

   A. respiratory disorders
   B. diabetes mellitus
   C. rheumatoid arthritis
   D. irritable bowel syndrome

8. The nurse will monitor the client receiving magnesium sulfate for the management of seizure disorder for which of the following indications of toxicity?

   A. hypotension
   B. tachypnea
   C. red man syndrome
   D. reddish orange urine

9. The most appropriate site for the nurse to administer diazepam intramuscularly is

   A. dorsal gluteal
   B. vastus lateralis
   C. deltoid
   D. ventral gluteal

10. When administering phenytoin, the nurse will

    A. administer intravenous forms of phenytoin with dextrose solutions
    B. avoid administration of intravenous phenytoin via a central venous access device
    C. administer enteral doses of phenytoin with a client's tube feeding
    D. turn a client's tube feeding off for at least 1 hour prior and 1 hour after the phenytoin suspension is administered

Multiple Response

Circle the best answers for each of the following questions. More than one answer is correct.

1. When working with clients receiving phenytoin therapy, the nurse will do which of the following? Select all that apply.

   A. Assess for the development of gingival hyperplasia.
   B. Encourage the client to perform oral hygiene.
   C. Teach the client to avoid any foods containing folic acid.
   D. Teach the client that this drug can decrease the effectiveness of oral contraceptives.
   E. Administer phenytoin with enteral feedings.
   F. Mix parenteral preparations of phenytoin with dextrose.

2. A new nurse is administering medications to a client for the management of seizure disorder. Which actions by the nurse require the supervising nurse to intervene? Select all that apply.

   A. Uses the deltoid site for intramuscular administration of acetazolamide.
   B. Questions the use of clonazepam for the treatment of a client with a history of chronic obstructive pulmonary disease.
   C. Informs the client taking felbamate to avoid unnecessary exposure to the sun.
   D. Assesses the cardiac monitor for the client receiving magnesium sulfate.
   E. Administers oxcarbazepine with valporic acid.
   F. Teaches the client to chew capsules of valporic acid.

Critical Thinking Exercises

1. List the major types of medications used to treat clients with seizure disorders, and describe their effects and contraindications.

2. Create a teaching plan for a client taking anticonvulsant medications, including focusing on ways to maintain client safety.

3. Identify nursing responsibilities associated with care of a client with a seizure disorder.

4. Investigate current and future trends in the management of clients with seizure disorders.

CHAPTER 32 *Substance Abuse*

Objectives

After reading Chapter 32 of *Pharmacological Aspects of Nursing Care,* 8th edition, the student will be able to:

1. Define the terms *substance misuse, substance abuse, habituation, physical dependence, psychological dependence, addiction, tolerance, cross-tolerance,* and *alcoholism.*

2. Explain the major pharmacological effects and usual method of abuse for each of the following substances:

    Club drugs

    Opiate and opiate-like drugs

    Sedative/hypnotics

    Alcohol

    Anxiolytics

    Amphetamine and amphetamine-like drugs

    Cocaine

    Cannabis

    Psychedelic drugs

    Tobacco

    Inhalants

3. Discuss appropriate ways by which dependency or abuse of each substance listed can be managed.

4. Explain the use of buprenorphine treatment, methadone maintenance, and narcotic antagonist therapy in the treatment of the opiate abuser.

5. Discuss appropriate nursing assessment for persons who abuse substances.

6. Describe the emergency nursing care given to substance abusers.

7. Apply the nursing process for persons who are chronic or recurrent substance abusers.

8. Discuss the management of health care workers who are substance abusers.

9. Describe several resources for information on substance abuse.

10. Successfully complete the games and activities in the online student StudyWARE.

Definitions

Supply the definitions for the following terms.

1. addiction _____

2. psychological dependence _____

3. tolerance _____

4. physical dependence _____

5. cross-tolerance _____

6. psychedelic drug _____

Fill in the Blank

Write in the missing information.

1. _____ is a pattern of repeated substance use in which a person feels better when using the substance than when not using it.

2. _____ is the reduced effect from the use of a substance resulting from its repeated use.

3. Two drugs used in the management of opiate dependence are _____ and _____.

4. _____ is the oldest psychoactive drug known.

5. The dependency of nurses on drugs is _____ than in the general population.

6. The four most dangerous components of smoke are _____, _____, _____, and_____.

Multiple Choice

Circle the best answer for each of the following questions. There is only one answer to each question.

1. A nurse is providing teaching to a local community group. The nurse identifies which of the the following as the two most commonly abused drugs?

   A. alcohol and nicotine
   B. alcohol and marijuana
   C. nicotine and narcotics
   D. narcotics and alcohol

2. The nurse expects which of the following drugs to be used in the treatment of a client who is dependent on opioids?

   A. secobarbitol
   B. methaqualone
   C. buprenophine
   D. lorazepam

3. The nurse teaches a community group that the most common infection seen in individuals who are intravenous drug users is

   A. severe streptococcal infections
   B. hepatitis B
   C. staphylococcal infections
   D. herpes simplex type I

4. What is the predominant pharmacologic effect of alcohol on the body?

   A. depressed central nervous system
   B. depressed cardiovascular system
   C. stimulated respiratory system
   D. stimulated gastrointestinal system

5. The nurses teaches the client that methadone maintenance programs usually last

   A. 1 week
   B. 1 month
   C. 1 year
   D. an indefinite period of time

6. Which of the following drugs does the nurse identify as an opioid?

   A. cocaine
   B. lysergic acid diethylamide
   C. dilaudid
   D. phencyclidine

7. Use of which of the following drugs most often causes damage to the nasal mucosa?

   A. pentobarbitol
   B. cocaine
   C. methaqualone
   D. mescaline

8. The nurse identifies which of the following drugs as producing flashbacks months or years after use?

   A. methylphenidate
   B. cocaine
   C. methamphetamine
   D. lysergic acid diethylamide (LSD)

9. When assessing a client who has smoked marijuana in moderation, the nurse expects to find

   A. alertness
   B. agitation
   C. ataxia
   D. aggressiveness

10. Clients who use cannibis in unusually large doses develop which of the following?

A. tolerance
B. physical dependence
C. heroine addiction
D. antisocial behavior

Multiple Response

Circle the best answers for each of the following questions. More than one answer is correct.

1. The nurse should teach clients using nicotine patches or gum about which of the following toxic effects? Select all that apply.

A. nausea
B. vomiting
C. dry mouth
D. constipation
E. dizziness
F. CNS stimulation

2. Which of the following statements about impaired health care workers does the nurse identify as true? Select all that apply.

A. The rate of drug dependency of nurses is approximately twice as great as that of the general population.
B. If drug abuse is suspected, the performance of the health care worker should be documented.
C. Counseling has not been found to be effective for health care workers who abuse substances.
D. If an employer suspects drug abuse, their first action should be to call the local police.
E. If a nurse abuses drugs, his or her license is immediately taken away.
F. Impaired nurses who refuse treatment should be reported to the State Board of Nursing.

Critical Thinking Exercises

1. Research the agents identified in this chapter that may cause physical or psychological dependence or addiction, along with the current treatments for chemical dependence on these agents.

2. Visit a drug rehabilitation facility and discuss with a licensed counselor the effects of barbiturates, amphetamines, depressants, opioids, and hallucinogens that brought clients to the facility.

3. Create a care plan for a client experiencing withdrawal symptoms, including educational materials.

CHAPTER 33 *Agents Affecting the Autonomic Nervous System*

Objectives

After reading Chapter 33 of *Pharmacological Aspects of Nursing Care,* 8th edition, the student will be able to:

1. Explain the major functions of the sympathetic and parasympathetic branches of the autonomic nervous system (ANS).
2. Identify the location and function of the alpha- and beta-adrenergic receptors.
3. Differentiate among and compare the actions of four categories of drugs that affect the ANS.
4. Discuss the mechanism of action of anticholinergic and direct-acting ANS agents.
5. Identify the conditions in which the use of ANS agents would be indicated or contraindicated.
6. Describe drug interactions and adverse effects of ANS agents.
7. Apply the nursing process relative to caring for clients receiving ANS drugs.
8. Successfully complete the games and activities in the online student StudyWARE.

Definitions

Supply the definitions for the following terms.

1. neurotransmitters _____
2. parasympathetic _____
3. somatic nervous system _____
4. sympathetic _____
5. ganglion _____
6. alpha$_1$ receptors _____
7. alpha$_2$ receptors _____
8. sympatholytics _____
9. beta$_1$-adrenergic receptors _____
10. beta$_2$-adrenergic receptors _____
11. "fight or flight" system _____
12. beta$_3$-adrenergic receptors _____

Fill in the Blank

Write in the missing information.

1. Cholinergic drugs mimic the actions of the *parasympathetic* nervous system.
2. The autonomic nervous system (ANS) has two divisions: the _____ and _____ branches.
3. Sympathomimetics utilize *catecholamines* to transmit messages.
4. A positive inotropic effect causes the heart rate to _____.
5. Sympathetic stimulation of the eye causes the pupil to *dilate*.
6. Most drugs with antispasmodic activity act by antagonizing the action of _____ at the postganglionic receptors in the parasympathetic nervous system.

7. _____ is an antispasmodic synthetic anticholinergic contraindicated in the treatment of clients with a history of myasthenia gravis.

8. Atropine sulfate and glycopyrrolate are frequently used preoperatively to decrease the risk for _____ and _____ during induction and maintenance of general anesthesia.

9. The most common cholinergic drugs used for the management of myasthenia gravis are _____, _____, and _____.

10. Adrenergic blockers cause blood vessels to _____.

Multiple Choice

Circle the best answer for each of the following questions. There is only one answer to each question.

1. It is most important for the nurse to assess the client taking anticholinergics for the development of which adverse effect?
   A. dry mouth
   B. ototoxicity
   C. increased urinary output
   D. diaphoresis

2. The nurse identifies which of the following as the antidote for adverse effects associated with anticholinergic agents?
   A. calcium gluconate
   B. naloxone
   C. epinephrine
   D. atropine sulfate

3. The nurse would question administration of an anticholinergic agent for the treatment of a client with a history of
   A. asthma
   B. reflex neurogenic bladder
   C. Parkinson's disease
   D. glaucoma

4. Which of the following medications would the nurse question in the treatment of a client with myasthenia gravis?
   A. scopolamine
   B. pyridostigmine
   C. edrophonium
   D. neostigmine

5. Normal antispasmodic doses of anticholinergic drugs are indicated in the treatment of
   A. narrow-angle glaucoma
   B. bronchial asthma
   C. benign prostatic hypertrophy
   D. overactive bladder

6. When a client receives high doses of anticholinergics, it is most important for the nurse to monitor the client for the development of
   A. tachycardia
   B. hypertension
   C. diaphoresis
   D. hyperthermia

7. The nurse identifies which agent as most likely to be used in the treatment of a client with Raynaud's disease?
   A. sympatholytics
   B. sympathomimetics
   C. parasympathomimetics
   D. parasympatholytics

8. Beta$_3$-adrenergic agonists have been found to be effective in the treatment of
   A. malnutrition
   B. diabetes mellitus Type 2
   C. diabetes insipidus
   D. glaucoma

9. The nurse identifies which of the following synthetic anticholinergics as contraindicated in the treatment of a client with a history of an obstructive gastrointestinal disorder?
   A. darifenacin
   B. dicyclomine
   C. oxybutynin chloride
   D. solifenacin succinate

10. Older clients taking cholinergics should be assessed by the nurse for the development of
   A. constipation
   B. diarrhea
   C. fluid retention
   D. hallucinations

Multiple Response

Circle the correct answers for each of the following questions. More than one answer is correct.

1. Which statements by a client taking an anticholinergic agent indicate that teaching has been effective? Select all that apply.

   A. Flushed skin is an indication that the medication needs to be stopped.
   B. I will call the health care provider if I have difficulty urinating.
   C. This medication will cause me to experience diarrhea.
   D. I will chew gum or suck on hard candy if my mouth is dry.
   E. I can expect to have blurred vision when starting this drug, but it will go away with time.
   F. If I experience heart palpitations, I will call my health care provider.

2. Organ responses to sympathetic stimulation include which of the following? Select all that apply.

   A. contraction of pupils
   B. dilation of bronchioles
   C. increased heart rate
   D. decreased force of heart contraction
   E. increased glycogenolysis
   F. contraction of the uterus

Critical Thinking Exercises

1. Discuss nursing responsibilities associated with use of cholinergics, anticholinergics, antispasmodics, and sympathomimetic medications, along with their uses and mechanisms of action. Provide two examples of each.

   _____

   _____

   _____

   _____

2. Describe adverse effects of cholinergics, anticholinergics, antispasmodics, and sympathomimetic medications.

   _____

   _____

   _____

   _____

3. Create a care plan for a client taking antispasmodics, including interventions and evaluation of goals.

   _____

   _____

   _____

   _____

CHAPTER 34 *Agents Affecting Thyroid, Parathyroid, and Pituitary Function*

Objectives

After reading Chapter 34 of *Pharmacological Aspects of Nursing Care,* 8th edition, the student will be able to:

1. Describe the mechanism by which thyroid hormones are synthesized in the body.
2. Discuss symptoms that may accompany hyperthyroidism and hypothyroidism.
3. Describe the mechanism by which each of the following forms of therapy relieves symptoms of hyperthyroidism: antithyroid drugs, iodides, radioactive iodine (I 131), beta-adrenergic blocking agents, and surgery.
4. Compare the causes, symptoms, and treatment of hypoparathyroidism and hyperparathyroidism.
5. Compare the causes, symptoms, and therapy of hypopituitarism, hyperpituitarism, and diabetes insipidus.
6. Discuss the factors that should be included in the teaching plan for clients undergoing drug therapy for diseases of the thyroid, parathyroid, and pituitary glands.
7. Discuss thyroid storm and distinguish its treatment from that of other thyroid conditions.
8. Discuss drug interactions and adverse effects of agents used to treat health alterations of the thyroid, parathyroid, and pituitary.
9. Apply the nursing process related to caring for clients receiving therapy for diseases of the thyroid, parathyroid, or pituitary gland.
10. Successfully complete the games and activities in the online student StudyWARE.

Definitions

Supply the definitions for the following terms.

1. hyperthyroidism _____
2. euthyroid _____
3. hypothyroidism _____
4. parathyroid gland _____
5. hypoparathyroidism _____
6. pituitary gland _____
7. acromegaly _____
8. diabetes insipidus _____

Fill in the Blank

Write in the missing information.

1. Typical clinical symptoms of hyperthyroidism include weight loss frequently accompanied by _____, _____, _____, _____, _____, _____, _____, _____, _____, _____, _____, and _____.
2. _____ and _____ are two chemically related antithyroid drugs that are effective in the management and control of hyperthyroidism.
3. _____ have been successfully used in suppressing some of the signs and symptoms of hyperthyroidism.

4. _____ is the drug most often associated with the development of drug-induced hyperthyroidism.

5. The most common form of hyperthyroidism is _____.

6. Clients with hypoparathyroidism usually have alterations of electrolyte balance including reduced serum _____ levels and elevated _____ levels.

7. Two of the most dramatic results of overproduction include _____ and _____.

8. The most effective therapy for diabetes insipidus is _____.

Multiple Choice

Circle the best answer for each of the following questions. There is only one answer to each question.

1. The synthesis of thyroid hormone is controlled by the
  A. hypothalamus
  B. anterior pituitary
  C. posterior pituitary
  D. thyroid

2. The release of thyroid stimulating hormone (TSH) is controlled by
  A. negative feedback
  B. positive feedback
  C. the autonomic nervous system (ANS)
  D. the central nervous system (CNS)

3. Which of the following medications does the nurse expect to be used in the treatment of hyperthyroidism?
  A. propylthiouracil
  B. levothyroxine sodium
  C. liothyronine sodium
  D. liotrix

4. A nurse is administering liothyronine sodium and levothyroxine sodium to a client. These medications are used to treat
  A. pituitary tumors
  B. hyperthyroidism
  C. hypothyroidism
  D. hypertension

5. A client presents with acute hypoparathyroidism. The nurse anticipates the administration of which medication to treat this condition?
  A. sodium chloride
  B. potassium chloride
  C. calcium chloride
  D. magnesium citrate

6. The nurses expects to find which of the following upon assessment of a client with diabetes insipidus?
  A. anuria
  B. polydipsia
  C. edema
  D. hyponatremia

7. A new nurse is administering potassium iodide to a client. Which action by the nurse requires the supervising nurse to intervene?
  A. Dilutes the medication with fruit juice.
  B. Has the client use a straw to take the medication.
  C. Dilutes the medication with milk.
  D. Holds the medication if client complains of a metallic taste in the mouth.

8. Hyperpituitarism may result in which of the following conditions?
  A. dwarfism
  B. hypernatremia
  C. short stature
  D. giantism

9. A client has vasopressin levels that are too high. Which finding does the nurse expect?
  A. polyuria
  B. constipation
  C. diuresis
  D. water intoxication

10. Which medication does the nurse identify as an effective treatment for Paget's disease?
  A. etidronate disodium
  B. somatropin
  C. adrenocorticotropic hormone (ACTH)
  D. desmopressin acetate

Multiple Response

Circle the best answers for each of the following questions. More than one answer is correct.

1. The nurse identifies which of the following as toxic signs and symptoms associated with hyperthyroidism? Select all that apply.

   A. restlessness
   B. weight loss
   C. hypoglycemia
   D. bradycardia
   E. nervousness
   F. excessive perspiration

2. Which of the following will the nurse include when teaching a client how to take thyroid replacement medication? Select all that apply.

   A. Take your pulse for 1 minute before taking the medication.
   B. Do not take the medication if your pulse is over 70.
   C. Take the medication in the evening.
   D. Call the health care provider if you experience insomnia.
   E. Call the health care provider if you experience excessive perspiration.
   F. Keep track of your weight.

Critical Thinking Exercises

1. Develop a teaching plan for clients with disorders of the thyroid gland.

2. Summarize nurse responsibilities associated with care of a client with disorders of the parathyroid gland.

3. Compare and contrast nursing responsibilities associated with care of a client experiencing disorders of the pituitary gland.

4. Describe the acute nursing interventions required for clients experiencing hyperthyroidism, hypothyroidism, hypoparathyroidism, hyperparathyroidism, hypopituitarism, hyperpituitarism, and diabetes insipidus.

CHAPTER 35 *Agents Used to Treat Hyperglycemia and Hypoglycemia*

Objectives

After reading Chapter 35 of *Pharmacological Aspects of Nursing Care,* 8th edition, the student will be able to:

1. Explain four functions of insulin in the body.
2. Discuss three adverse effects associated with insulin administration.
3. Identify the generic and brand names of insulins currently in use.
4. Describe the mechanism of action of oral hypoglycemic agents.
5. Discuss adverse effects commonly associated with the use of sulfonylurea oral hypoglycemic agents.
6. Discuss the pancreatic hormones used in treating hypoglycemia and hyperglycemia.
7. Differentiate among short-, intermediate-, and long-acting insulins and give an example of each.
8. Discuss the nursing assessment of a person with diabetes mellitus.
9. Distinguish the signs and symptoms of insulin reaction from those of diabetic ketoacidosis.
10. Compare the treatment of insulin reaction and ketoacidosis.
11. Explain in a stepwise fashion the procedures used in mixing and administering insulins.
12. Discuss the sites commonly used for insulin administration and plan a rotation pattern.
13. Discuss the local tissue responses possible with repeated insulin injections.
14. Explain common drug interactions associated with the use of oral antidiabetic agents.
15. Discuss three factors that may produce a change in a diabetic client's insulin requirement.
16. Briefly describe how a sliding scale of insulin administration works and describe the use of insulin pumps.
17. Differentiate between open- and closed-loop insulin pumps.
18. Apply the nursing process related to care of clients experiencing hypoglycemia or hyperglycemia.
19. Successfully complete the games and activities in the online student StudyWARE.

Definitions

Supply the definitions for the following terms.

1. diabetes mellitus _____
2. Type 1 diabetes mellitus _____
3. Type 2 diabetes mellitus _____
4. insulin glargine (Lantus) _____
5. continuous subcutaneous insulin infusion (CSII) _____
6. meglitinides _____
7. exenatide (Byetta) _____
8. U-100 _____

Fill in the Blank

Write in the missing information.

1. _diazoxide_ is a nondiuretic benzothiediazine agent used for the oral management of hypoglycemia.
2. Insulin mixtures should only be administered via the _SQ_ route.
3. Aspart insulin can be mixed with _NPH_ insulin.

4. Lispro insulin is stable when used in an external pump for _____48_____ hours.

5. _____Acarbose_____ should be administered with the first bite of food the client is receiving.

6. The duration of action of glimepiride (Amaryl) is _____24_____ hours.

7. Women taking _____Avandia_____ should be monitored for the development of fractures.

8. A common goal of clients in the management of diabetes mellitus is a hemoglobin A1c value of _____6_____.

Multiple Choice

Circle the best answer for each of the following questions. There is only one answer to each question.

1. The nurse will discard which type of insulin if it is cloudy?
   A. lente
   B. NPH
   C. lispro
   D. ultralente

2. Which agent used to treat hyperglycemia does the nurse associate with an increased incidence of pancreatitis?
   A. exenatide (Byetta)
   B. miglitol (Glyset)
   C. piglitazone (Actos)
   D. nateglinide (Starlix)

3. The nurse should assesses clients taking which class of oral hypoglycemics for the development of syndrome of inappropriate antidiuretic hormone (SIADH)?
   A. glitazones
   B. meglitinides
   C. sulfonureas
   D. alpha-glucosidases inhibitors

4. When working with clients taking oral hypoglycemic agents, the nurse monitors for edema and worsening heart failure for clients taking
   A. glipizide (Glucotrol)
   B. metformin HCl (Glucophage)
   C. rosiglitazone (Avandia)
   D. miglitol (Glyset)

5. The nurse identifies which type of insulin as having the most rapid onset of action?
   A. insulin aspart
   B. regular
   C. NPH
   D. glargine

6. When drawing up insulin that needs to be mixed for administration, in which order is the insulin drawn up?
   A. long-acting, then short-acting insulin
   B. regular, then lente insulin
   C. ultralente, then intermediate-acting insulin
   D. order doesn't matter

7. The nurse will administer subcutaneous insulin at an angle of how many degrees?
   A. 50
   B. 45
   C. 75
   D. 90

8. After mixing lispro and ultralente insulin, the insulin should be administered within how many minutes?
   A. 5
   B. 15
   C. 40
   D. 60

9. If a nurse finds a client who is a known diabetic in an unconscious state, the standard of care is to initially treat the client for
   A. hyperglycemia
   B. diabetic ketoacidosis
   C. hypoglycemia
   D. hypernatremia

10. When teaching a client about the administration of insulin, which of the following comments made by the client would indicate that more teaching is needed?
    A. "I have to insert the same amount of air into the insulin vial as the amount of insulin I need to withdraw."
    B. "I don't understand why I can't take my insulin in a pill like my grandfather does."
    C. "When using my abdomen for my insulin injection, I need to leave at least 1–2 inches from my belly button free from injections."
    D. "I should monitor my blood sugar before meals and before I go to bed at night."

Multiple Response

Circle the best answers for each of the following questions. More than one answer is correct.

1. When providing teaching for a client who is a Type 2 diabetic, which of the following will the nurse include? Select all that apply.
   A. There is no cure for diabetes.
   B. Medication therapy is the mainstay of treatment.
   C. You may temporarily need insulin injections if you have surgery.
   D. It is possible to control the disease.
   E. You may temporarily need insulin injections if you experience emotional stress.
   F. You will not develop complications like a person with Type 1 diabetes does.

2. When teaching a client about insulin therapy, which of the following will the nurse include? Select all that apply.
   A. Place the needle of the syringe at a 60-degree angle to the skin.
   B. If you pull back on the syringe after the needle is in the skin and there is blood, do not inject the insulin.
   C. Use your calf for injection of insulin.
   D. Wipe the area where you will inject the needle with an antiseptic and allow it to dry before inserting the needle.
   E. Withdraw the clear insulin first, then the cloudy.
   F. Use a needle that is 5/8-inch or shorter.

Critical Thinking Exercises

1. Develop a chart representing the various types of insulin therapy, reviewing associated nursing responsibilities associated with each type of insulin.

2. Develop a teaching plan for a client with Type 1 diabetes mellitus and one for a client with Type 2 diabetes mellitus. Compare and contrast information presented to the clients.

3. Develop a chart comparing and contrasting various oral hypoglycemic agents used in the treatment of hyperglycemia, focusing on nursing responsibilities associated with each drug.

4. Practice administration of single-dose and mixed insulins.

_____

_____

_____

_____

CHAPTER 36 *Sex Hormones*

Objectives

After reading Chapter 36 of *Pharmacological Aspects of Nursing Care,* 8th edition, the student will be able to:

1. Describe the classes of sex hormones and give an example of an agent in each class.
2. Discuss estrogens and progestins commonly employed in hormonal drug products.
3. Discuss common adverse effects associated with the use of estrogens and progestational agents.
4. Describe five therapeutic uses for estrogens.
5. Describe five therapeutic uses for progestational agents.
6. Explain the mechanism(s) by which estrogens and progestins act to prevent conception.
7. Describe the usual method of administration for "combination" and "minipill" types of oral contraceptives.
8. Describe the difference between monophasic, biphasic, and triphasic combination oral contraceptive products.
9. Explain the mechanism by which clomiphene citrate, human chorionic gonadotropin (HCG), menotropins, and gonadorelin acetate act as ovulation stimulants.
10. Identify and discuss two common adverse effects associated with the use of ovulation stimulants.
11. Describe five therapeutic uses for androgens.
12. Discuss erectile dysfunction and the agents used to treat this disorder.
13. Discuss the therapeutic use(s) of androgen hormone inhibitors.
14. Discuss the therapeutic uses and adverse effects associated with the use of anabolic agents.
15. Apply the nursing process for clients receiving long-term treatment with sex hormones.
16. Describe the content of an instructional program for women taking oral contraceptives.
17. Successfully complete the games and activities in the online student StudyWARE.

Definitions

Supply the definitions for the following terms.

1. androgen _____
2. estrogen and progesterone _____
3. diethylstilbestrol (DES) _____
4. erectile dysfunction _____

Fill in the Blank

Write in the missing information.

1. When clients take estrogens, they may require upward adjustments of _____ and _____ drug dosages and a reduction of _____.
2. When one or two tablets of an oral contraceptive have been missed, the client should be advised to use an additional means of contraception for _____.
3. Clients on prolonged estrogen therapy should have their blood pressure checked periodically and be assessed for the development of _____.
4. If _____ symptoms develop during clomiphene citrate therapy, it is discontinued.
5. Anabolic agents used in excess are associated with a higher incidence of _____ at relatively young ages.

Multiple Choice

Circle the best answer for each of the following questions. There is only one answer to each question.

1. It is most important for the nurse to assess a client receiving estrogen therapy for the development of

   A. pregnancy
   B. stroke
   C. thromboembolism
   D. hormonal dysfunction

2. Which of the following medications often requires an upward adjustment when administered with estrogen?

   A. corticosteroids
   B. antidiabetics
   C. bronchodilators
   D. diuretics

3. Which of the following drugs is used to decrease the size of the prostate in men with symptomatic benign prostatic hypertrophy (BPH)?

   A. dutasteride (Adovart)
   B. tamsulosin HCl (Flomax)
   C. vardenafil (Levitra)
   D. tadalafil (Cialis)

4. The consistent inability to obtain and maintain an erection sufficient for sexual intercourse is called

   A. libido
   B. erectile dysfunction
   C. psychosomatic
   D. potency

5. Which of the following drugs remains in effect for the longest period of time?

   A. sildenafil citrate (Viagra)
   B. vardenafil (Levitra)
   C. tadalafil (Cialis)
   D. alvimil

6. The nurse identifies which of the following statements about testosterone as being true?

   A. It exerts a catabolic effect.
   B. It is administered intravenously.
   C. It is used primarily for the treatment of hypogonadism.
   D. It is not used in females.

7. The nurse anticipates use of which of the following drugs for the treatment of endometriosis?

   A. medroxyprogesterone acetate
   B. megestrol acetate
   C. norethindrone acetate
   D. progesterone

8. Which of the following drugs does the nurse identify as useful in supporting implantation of the embryo?

   A. progesterone
   B. estradiol
   C. norethindrone acetate
   D. megestrol acetate

9. It is most important for the nurse to assess the client taking medroxyprogesterone (Depo-Provera) for the development of

   A. restrictive airway disease
   B. hypoglycemia
   C. rash
   D. osteoporosis

10. The nurse should teach female children of women who took diethylstilbestrol (DES) that they are at an increased risk for the development of

    A. renal failure
    B. infertility
    C. osteosarcomas
    D. genitourinary abnormalities

Multiple Response

Circle the best answers for each of the following questions. More than one answer is correct.

1. Which of the following will the nurse include when teaching a client taking oral contraceptives and estrogen replacement therapy? Select all that apply.

    A. Perform a monthly breast self-exam.
    B. Yearly Pap testing is no longer needed.
    C. Condoms should be used to prevent sexually transmitted disease.
    D. If you develop breakthrough bleeding, stop taking the medication.
    E. If you experience nausea, stop taking the medication.
    F. Your menstrual flow may decrease in amount and is no cause for concern.

2. Which of the following statements about use of drugs to treat benign prostatic hypertrophy indicates that more teaching is indicated? Select all that apply.

    A. Dutasteride (Adovart) is used to increase the flow of urine.
    B. Tamsulosin HCl (Flomax) is used to decrease the size of the prostate.
    C. Finasteride (Proscar) is used to decrease the size of the prostate.
    D. I will not donate blood for 6 months after the last dose of the medication.
    E. Because my partner is of childbearing age, I will use barrier protection while taking this medication.
    F. A result of taking this medication should be improved urinary flow.

Critical Thinking Exercises

1. Discuss the role of sex hormones in the development and maturation of the human body.

    _____

    _____

    _____

    _____

2. Create a teaching plan for a client taking oral contraceptive agents, including nursing interventions. Specify techniques for promoting client safety.

    _____

    _____

    _____

    _____

3. Develop a care plan for a client taking medications to treat erectile dysfunction.

    _____

    _____

    _____

    _____

4. Develop a teaching plan for a client taking medications for benign prostatic hypertrophy.

_____

_____

_____

_____

CHAPTER 37 Agents Used in Obstetrical Care

Objectives

After reading Chapter 37 of *Pharmacological Aspects of Nursing Care,* 8th edition, the student will be able to:

1. Describe the classifications of agents most commonly used in obstetrical care and give an example of each class.
2. Discuss the therapeutic uses of oxytocic agents.
3. Explain why the action of oxytocin increases during the last several weeks before term.
4. Discuss the desired actions, side effects, and usual modes of administering the agents commonly used in labor and delivery.
5. Describe several agents secreted in breastmilk.
6. Discuss appropriate areas for assessment in women receiving pharmacological agents as part of their obstetrical care.
7. Apply the nursing process related to caring for clients receiving agents to promote labor and delivery, agents to control postpartum hemorrhage, uterine relaxants for the treatment of preterm labor, and agents to induce abortion.
8. Successfully complete the games and activities in the online student StudyWARE.

Definitions

Supply the definitions for the following terms.

1. oxytocic agents _selective stimulants of uterine smooth muscle_
2. bromocriptine mesylate (Parlodel) _agent used to supress lactation_
3. ergot alkaloid _agent used to stimulate uterine smooth muscle_
4. ritodrine HCl _inhibits uterine smooth muscle contraction, prolongs gestation_
5. terbutaline sulfate (Brethine) _stimulates beta2 receptors in uterus, thus relaxing the uterus_

Fill in the Blank

Write in the missing information.

1. Normal fetal heart rate is considered to be ___120___ to ___160___ beats/min.
2. ___Cervidil___ is a drug often used to ripen the cervix prior to oxytocin-induced labor.
3. Following delivery ___Methergine___ may be administered to increase uterine tone and to decrease postpartum bleeding.
4. When dinoprostone (Prostin E2) is used intravaginally, the nurse should be aware that ___fever___ may occur.
5. Maternal hypotension resulting from terbutaline therapy is treated by encouraging the woman to lie on her ___left___ side.

Multiple Choice

Circle the best answer for each of the following questions. There is only one answer to each question.

1. A client is experiencing extensive uterine bleeding after delivery. The nurse anticipates administration of which of the following drugs?
   A. Rho(D) immune globulin
   B. methylergonovine maleate (Methergine)
   C. oxytocin (Pitocin)
   D. ritodrine HCl

Back of Books...

2. The nurse identifies which of the following drugs as an oxytocic agent?

   A. terbutaline
   B. ritodrine HCl

   C. dinoprostone
   D. oxytocin

3. The nurse administers dinoprostone to a client to cause what effect?

   A. relax the uterus
   B. stimulate the uterus to contract

   C. prolong the gestational period
   D. suppress lactation

4. The nurse anticipates administration of which drug to inhibit preterm labor?

   A. terbutaline sulfate
   B. oxytocin

   C. Rh0(D) immune globulin
   D. methylergonovine maleate

   Back of book says A, mag sulfate?

5. This medication is a gel used to ripen the cervix of a woman having an induced labor.

   A. terbutaline sulfate
   B. methylergonovine maleate

   C. ritodrine HCl
   D. dinoprostone

6. Which statement by a client receiving uterine relaxants for the treatment of preterm labor indicates more teaching is indicated?

   A. "I will limit my physical activity to that prescribed."
   B. "I will avoid sexual intercourse."
   C. "I will avoid orgasm."
   D. "I will start to prepare my breasts for lactation 3 weeks before my due date."

7. The nurse identifies which of the following as a possible side effect to bromocriptine mesylate (Parlodel) therapy?

   A. hypertension
   B. rash

   C. increased vaginal bleeding
   D. dizziness

8. Which statement by the client indicates that more teaching about lactation suppression is indicated?

   A. "I will wear a snug bra at all times except when I bathe."
   B. "I will avoid warm soaks to my breasts."
   C. "I will not express any milk from my breasts."
   D. "If I experience discomfort in my breasts, I will take aspirin."

9. A client has received mifepristone. It is most important for the nurse to assess the client for the development of which of the following?

   A. infection
   B. rash

   C. high blood sugar
   D. impaired renal function

10. The nurse identifies which of the following statements about Rho(D) immune globulin (RhoGAM) as being true?

   A. It is obtained from the serum of cows.
   B. It is administered via the intravenous route.
   C. It must be administered to the mother within 72 hours of delivery.
   D. It should be administered to the infant within 24 hours of delivery.

Multiple Response

Circle the best answers for each of the following questions. More than one answer is correct.

1. Which of the following statements about Rho(D) immune globulin (RhoGAM) does the nurse identify as being true? Select all that apply.

   A. It should be stored in the refrigerator before use.
   B. It should not be allowed to freeze.
   C. Adverse effects of the drug are frequent and severe.
   D. It is administered to nonsensitized Rh-negative mothers after delivery of an Rh-positive infant.
   E. It provides protection against erythroblastosis fetalis.
   F. It should be taken by the mother by mouth for 1 week twice daily with food.

2. Which of the following will the nurse include when teaching the client about bromocriptine mesylate (Parlodel) therapy? Select all that apply.

   A. Rise slowly from a sitting to a standing position.
   B. Do not take the drug for more than 7 days.
   C. If you experience discomfort in your breasts, ibuprofen may be used.
   D. Pack ice around your breasts throughout the day for the first 3 days after delivery.
   E. If your breasts swell, stimulate the nipples to allow the milk to be released.
   F. Avoid use of warm soaks on your breasts.

Critical Thinking Exercises

1. Develop a teaching plan for a client receiving oxytocic agents.

   _____

   _____

   _____

   _____

2. Develop a chart comparing and contrasting nursing interventions associated with oxytocic agents.

   _____

   _____

   _____

   _____

3. Develop a teaching plan for a client in preterm labor receiving uterine relaxants.

   _____

   _____

   _____

   _____

4. Summarize methods used for termination of pregnancy.

   _____

   _____

   _____

   _____

CHAPTER 38 *Agents That Affect Immunity*

Objectives

After reading Chapter 38 of *Pharmacological Aspects of Nursing Care,* 8th edition, the student will be able to:

1. Differentiate the drugs most often used to stimulate the immune system from those used to suppress the immune system.
2. List the recommended childhood immunizations.
3. List the recommended immunizations for adults.
4. Explain the major components of the immune system.
5. Discuss the major adverse effects and drug interactions of drugs used to suppress the immune system.
6. Apply the nursing process for clients receiving drugs to stimulate the immune system.
7. Apply the nursing process for clients receiving drugs to suppress the immune system.
8. Successfully complete the games and activities in the online student StudyWARE.

Definitions

Supply the definitions for the following terms.

1. vaccine _____
2. active immunization _____
3. interferons and interleukins _____
4. immunosuppressants _____
5. cyclosporin _____

Fill in the Blank

Write in the missing information.

1. _____ is the study of the molecules, cells, and organs responsible for the recognition and disposal of foreign materials, how those materials interact, and how their action can be diminished or enhanced.
2. _____ enhances or stimulates the body's own immune system to dramatically increase the body's resistance to certain infections.
3. The muscle spasms associated with a bite by a black widow spider are treated with _____ and the pain is treated with _____.
4. BCG vaccine is a _____ vaccine that must be treated carefully.
5. Before administering the measles (rubeola) vaccine to a client, the nurse should assess for client allergy to _____ and _____.

Multiple Choice

Circle the best answer for each of the following questions. There is only one answer to each question.

1. A newborn is in jeopardy of developing hemolytic anemia. The nurse anticipates administration of
   A. Rho(D) immune globulin
   B. hepatitis B immune globulin
   C. immune globulin
   D. gamma globulin

2. A female client has received measles, mumps, and rubella vaccine, live (M-M-R II). The nurse will instruct the client to avoid pregnancy for

A. 1 week

B. 1 month

C. 2 months

D. 3 months

3. The nurse identifies which of the following agents as most effective in the prevention of organ rejection?

A. muromonab-CD3

B. sirolimus

C. daclizumab

D. cyclosporine

4. Before administering black widow spider species antivenin to a client, it is most important for the nurse to assess the client for an allergy to

A. shrimp

B. penicillin

C. eggs

D. horse serum

5. When working with a client who has a venomous snake bite, it is most important for the nurse to

A. encourage the client to walk

B. administer the antivenin within 6 hours of the bite

C. prepare the patient for amputation surgery

D. start hemodialysis

6. A client is ordered cyclosporine therapy. It is most important for the nurse to use caution if which of the following drugs is also ordered?

A. aminoglycosides

B. insulin

C. anticoagulants

D. digitalis

7. A client has been exposed to hepatitis B. The nurse identifies which of the following as the preferred route for administering hepatitis B immune globulin?

A. by mouth

B. subcutaneously

C. intravenously

D. intramuscularly

8. The nurse will administer the initial dose of cytomegalovirus (CMV) immune globulin _____ hours after transplant surgery.

A. 24

B. 36

C. 48

D. 72

Multiple Response

Circle the best answers for each of the following questions. More than one answer is correct.

1. When administering influenza virus vaccines, the nurse will do which of the following? Select all that apply.

A. Asses the client for development of Guillian-Barrè syndrome as an adverse effect.

B. Tell the client to immediately call the health care provider if experiencing malaise after the vaccine is administered.

C. Ask if the client is allergic to chicken eggs.

D. Use the deltoid site for administration.

E. Tell the client to go to the emergency department if he or she develops a red and indurated area at the injection site.

F. Defer administration if the client has an acute respiratory infection.

2. The nurse identifies which of the following statements about immunosuppressant agents as true? Select all that apply.

A. These agents are primarily used to prevent organ rejection.

B. They act by suppressing T lymphocytes.

C. An adverse effect of cyclosporine is gum hyperplasia.

D. Cyclosporin is available for parenteral use only.

E. Muromonab-CD3 works specifically against bacterial antigens.

F. Daclizumab destroys RNA of rejected organ tissue.

Critical Thinking Exercises

1. Design a teaching poster of the required precautions for a client who has undergone a bone marrow transplant.

   _____

   _____

   _____

   _____

2. Create a care plan for a client who had a heart transplant. Specify techniques for promoting pain relief and client safety.

   _____

   _____

   _____

   _____

3. Summarize nursing responsibilities associated with childhood immunizations.

   _____

   _____

   _____

   _____

4. Describe nursing responsibilities associated with adult immunizations.

   _____

   _____

   _____

   _____

CHAPTER 39 *Antineoplastic Agents and Adjunct Drugs Used in Cancer Treatment*

Objectives

After reading Chapter 39 of *Pharmacological Aspects of Nursing Care,* 8th edition, the student will be able to:

1. Describe the cell cycle and how it is affected by the use of antineoplastic agents.

2. Discuss the major classes of antineoplastic agents and give an example of an agent in each class.

3. Explain the major therapeutic actions, adverse effects, and drug interactions of each class of antineoplastic agents.

4. Describe important aspects of nursing assessment for clients receiving cancer chemotherapy.

5. Apply the nursing process for clients receiving antineoplastic agents.

6. Apply the nursing process for clients receiving each of the classes of antineoplastic agents.

7. Review general principles of nursing care for clients receiving therapy via tunneled catheters, and implanted vascular access devices and pumps (see Chapter 3).

8. Discuss measures taken to ensure the safe administration of antineoplastic agents.

9. Explain the role of the nurse in the care of clients receiving investigational agents.

10. Successfully complete the games and activities in the online student StudyWARE.

Definitions

Supply the definitions for the following terms.

1. cancer _____

2. antineoplastic agents _____

3. alkylating agents _____

4. adjuvant agents _____

5. monoclonial antibodies _____

6. biologic-response modifiers _____

7. miotic inhibitors _____

8. radioactive drugs _____

Fill in the Blank

Write in the missing information.

1. _____ is a synthetic version of erythropoietin that stimulates bone marrow to produce red blood cells.

2. _____ is a colony-stimulating factor used to increase the number of leukocytes after chemotherapy.

3. To prevent and control nausea and vomiting associated with chemotherapy, clients receive _____.

4. To prevent and treat oral mucositis associated with chemotherapy and radiation therapy for cancers, _____ has been found to be effective.

5. _____, or dry mouth, may occur as a result of treatment for cancer.

6. During the cell cycle, the cell goes through four phases or stages, _____, _____, _____, and _____.

Multiple Choice

Circle the best answer for each of the following questions. There is only one answer to each question.

1. The nurse identifies which of the following statements about mesna as being true?

   A. Mesna is used to rescue the lung from pulmonary toxicity.
   B. Mesna facilitates removal of uric acid from the body.
   C. Mesna is used to rescue the urinary bladder from potential hemorrhagic cystitis.
   D. Mesna is used to prevent cardiotoxicity.

2. For a client receiving doxorubicin HCl, it is most important for the nurse to assess the client for the development of

   A. cardiotoxicity
   B. neurotoxicity
   C. pulmonary toxicity
   D. ototoxicity

3. When administering cyclophosphamide to a client, it is most important for the nurse to assess the client for the development of

   A. cardiotoxicity
   B. neurotoxicity
   C. hemorrhagic cystitis
   D. ototoxicity

4. When administering predinsone by mouth to a client with cancer, the nurse will

   A. administer the drug on an empty stomach
   B. administer the medication at bedtime
   C. monitor the client for hyperglycemia
   D. avoid use of any anti-infective drugs

5. The nurse administers methotrexate and prepares to follow up with administration of which agent to neutralize the toxic effects of methotrexate on the hematologic system?

   A. mesna
   B. leucovorin
   C. pegfilgrastim
   D. ibuprofen

6. The nurse understands that the maintenance intravenous fluid infused before and after intravenous methotrexate is

   A. 10% dextrose/0.45% normal saline
   B. Lactated Ringer's solution
   C. 0.9% sodium chloride
   D. 5% dextrose and sodium bicarbonate

7. When teaching a client about paclitaxel therapy, the nurse will include which of the following statements?

   A. If you experience a headache, take acetaminophen.
   B. You should continue to take at least 2 tablets of aspirin a day.
   C. If your body aches, use ibuprofen to relieve the pain.
   D. The alopecia from use of this drug is permanent.

8. The nurse will teach the client receiving procarbazine HCl to avoid which of the following?

   A. bananas
   B. aged cheese
   C. chicken breast
   D. wheat bread

9. Which statement by the client who is receiving chemotherapy indicates teaching regarding nutritional needs has been effective?

   A. "I will eat three large meals a day and avoid snacking."
   B. "I will restrict the amount of protein I eat."
   C. "I will eat foods high in vitamin C."
   D. "I will only take medications for nausea and vomiting after I have vomited at least twice."

10. The nurse identifies the most common electrolyte disorder associated with peritoneal infusion of cisplatin as

   A. hypomagnesemia
   B. hyponatremia
   C. hypercalcemia
   D. hyperkalemia

Multiple Response

Circle the best answers for each of the following questions. More than one answer is correct.

1. When administering an antineoplastic drug into the peritoneal cavity, the nurse will do which of the following? Select all that apply.

    A. Dilute the antineoplastic drug in D5W.
    B. Warm the antineoplastic drug to body temperature.
    C. Have the client lie still for 1 hour.
    D. Ask the client to perform the Valsalva maneuver to facilitate fluid drainage.
    E. Maintain sterile technique.
    F. Following fluid drainage, flush the catheter with D5W.

2. When working with a client receiving chemotherapy, the nurse will do which of the following? Select all that apply.

    A. Institute bleeding precautions for a client with a platelet count of 40,000 cells/mm3.
    B. Inform the primary care provider if the client's oxygen saturation is 88.
    C. Monitor the intravenous site every hour during chemotherapy administration.
    D. If extravasation occurs, decrease the infusion rate of the chemotherapy by one half.
    E. Inform the client that the alopecia resulting from chemotherapy is permanent.
    F. Contact the health care provider if the client's urine pH is 4.0.

Critical Thinking Exercises

1. Review the cell cycle and identify the site at which various anticancer agents exert their effect.

    _____

    _____

    _____

    _____

2. Review nursing responsibilities associated with each type of drug used to treat clients with cancer.

    _____

    _____

    _____

    _____

3. Review the orientation manual used to educate nurses on the administration of drugs to treat clients with cancer at the facility where you have clinical experiences.

    _____

    _____

    _____

    _____

4. Review nursing responsibilities associated with use of adjuvant agents in the care of clients with cancer.

_____

_____

_____

_____

5. Collaborate with individuals in your class to develop appropriate teaching plans for clients with cancer receiving various treatment modalities. Share your findings.

_____

_____

_____

_____

CHAPTER 40 Agents Used in the Treatment of Conditions of the Eyes

Objectives

After reading Chapter 40 of *Pharmacological Aspects of Nursing Care,* 8th edition, the student will be able to:

1. Discuss four purposes for using mydriatic agents.
2. Describe two major classes of mydriatic agents, giving an example of each.
3. List the three classes of ophthalmic anti-infective agents, giving an example of each.
4. Discuss two purposes for using corticosteroid ophthalmic preparations.
5. Discuss the pathophysiology of glaucoma.
6. Distinguish between narrow- and wide-angle glaucoma.
7. Explain three classes of agents that decrease the formation of aqueous humor.
8. Explain two classes of agents that increase the outflow of aqueous humor.
9. Identify one class of agents that decreases the formation of aqueous humor and increases its outflow.
10. Apply in order the steps of the procedure for administering ophthalmic agents.
11. Apply the nursing process related to the administration of ophthalmic agents.
12. Successfully complete the games and activities in the online student StudyWARE.

Definitions

Supply the definitions for the following terms.

1. narrow-angle glaucoma _____
2. carbonic-anhydrase inhibitors _____
3. open-angle glaucoma _____
4. osmotic diuretics _____
5. sympathomimetic agents _____
6. miotics _____
7. cholinesterase inhibitors _____
8. beta-adrenergic blockers _____
9. natamycin _____
10. mydratic _____

Fill in the Blank

Write in the missing information.

1. Mydratic drugs cause the pupil to _____.
2. Miotic drugs cause the pupil to _____.
3. Paralysis of accommodation is called _____.
4. _____ is an agent that can be used in the treatment of fungal keratitis.
5. If viral infections of the eye are not treated effectively, they can result in_____.

6. Clients using corticosteroids in the eye should be closely monitored for the development of _____.

7. Glaucoma is characterized by the development of _____.

8. The most popular agent used to constrict the pupil is _____.

Multiple Choice

Circle the best answer for each of the following questions. There is only one answer to each question.

1. The nurse will include which of the following statements when teaching a client about epinephrine opthalmic solution?

   A. Wait 15 minutes before inserting a contact lens.
   B. It is normal for the solution to turn brown.
   C. Expect to see participates form in the solution.
   D. The medication must be stored in the refrigerator.

2. Which statement made by a client receiving cyclopentolate HCl indicates that more teaching is necessary?

   A. "The drug may burn when instilled."
   B. "A low heart rate is commonly found when people take this drug."
   C. "I should not drive after taking this drug because I may become disoriented."
   D. "I should wait 5 to 10 minutes before administering the second drop of this medication."

3. The nurse identifies which of the following statements about acetazolamide (Diamox) as being true?

   A. It may be used with miotics.
   B. It may not be used with mydriatics.
   C. It may cause a false positive test for blood in urine.
   D. Intravenous administration should be avoided.

4. Which of the following medications is most often used in the prevention of opthalmia neonatorum?

   A. tetracycline   C. erythromycin
   B. sulfacetamide   D. polymyxin B

5. Which of the following drugs does the nurse identify as contraindicated in the treatment of viral infections of the eye?

   A. corticosteroid   C. vidarabine
   B. idoxuridine   D. trifluridine

6. The nurse identifies which of the following as the drug of choice for the treatment of chlamydial infections?

   A. tobramycin   C. silver nitrate
   B. tetracycline   D. ciprofloxacin

7. Clients receiving timolol should be informed about potential drug interactions with what class of drugs?

   A. antidiabetics   C. cardiac drugs
   B. antimicrobials   D. opioids

8. The nurse should teach the client receiving mydriatics to

   A. not drive after nightfall
   B. expect to lose the ability to see color
   C. wear sunglasses to protect the eyes from light sensitivity
   D. identify darkening of the iris as a normal effect of this medication

9. When administering pilocarpine, it is most important for the nurse to assess the patient for a history of

   A. asthma   C. renal disease
   B. diabetes mellitus   D. hepatic failure

Multiple Response

Circle the best answers for each of the following questions. More than one answer is correct.

1. When administering an opthalmic preparation, the nurse will do which of the following? Select all that apply.

   A. Administer ointments into the lower lid.
   B. Only use agents that are labeled for topical use.
   C. Stop treatment once symptoms subside.
   D. Always apply an eye patch after administering cholinesterase inhibitors.
   E. Wash hands immediately before and after administering an eye medication.
   F. Warn the client that some eye medications cause some transient stinging of the eye.

2. When administering eyedrops, the nurse will do which of the following? Select all that apply.

   A. Document OS as the left eye.
   B. Inform the client that vision may be blurred temporarily.
   C. Document OU as both eyes.
   D. Ask the client to blink several times after the eyedrops have been administered.
   E. Document OD as right eye.
   F. Place the eyedrop on the pupil.

Critical Thinking Exercises

1. Create a presentation for clients on the major types of medications used for the treatment of glaucoma, and describe their effects and contraindications.

   _____

   _____

   _____

   _____

2. Create a teaching plan for a client taking miotics, mydriatics, prostaglandin-inhibiting agents, cholinesterase-inhibiting agents, osmotic diuretics, and beta-adrenergic agents. Include interventions and ways to maintain client safety.

   _____

   _____

   _____

   _____

3. Create a visual presentation, appropriate for client teaching, of the steps taken when administering eyedrops.

   _____

   _____

   _____

   _____s

CHAPTER 41 *Agents Used in the Treatment of Conditions of the Ears*

Objectives

After reading Chapter 41 of *Pharmacological Aspects of Nursing Care,* 8th edition, the student will be able to:

1. Explain the anatomical parts of the ear.
2. Discuss the three primary ear disorders which otic agents are used to treat.
3. Discuss otitis media and how it is treated with otic solutions.
4. Discuss the seven classifications of otic agents, providing an example of each.
5. Apply the nursing process related to the administration of otic agents.
6. Successfully complete the games and activities in the online student StudyWARE.

Definitions

Supply the definitions for the following terms.

1. middle ear _____
2. inner ear _____
3. cerumen _____
4. pinna _____
5. cochlea _____

Fill in the Blank

Write in the missing information.

1. The most common middle ear disorder is _____.
2. When compared to adults, the eustachian tubes in children are _____ and _____.
3. _____ are agents that can be used to loosen and assist in the removal of impacted cerumen.
4. _____ otic medications need to be administered via sterile procedure.
5. To administer eardrops, the pinna of the child should be pulled _____ and _____.

Multiple Choice

Circle the best answer for each of the following questions. There is only one answer to each question.

1. The nurse is administering benzocaine (Otocaine) to a client with otitis media. The nurse is aware that the effects of this medication include all of the following except
   A. pain relief
   B. relief of swelling
   C. relief of congestion
   D. anti-infective

2. When administering eardrop to a child, the nurse should
   A. pull the pinna up and back
   B. pull the pinna down and back
   C. Pull the pinna straight back
   D. have the child sit with the affected ear facing down

3. A client has an ear infection caused by *Proteus mirabilis.* The nurse anticipates treatment with which of the following?

A. gentamicin

B. ciprofloxacin

C. ofloxacin

D. Cortisporin

4. Which of the following indicate that treatment for a client with otitis media has been effective? The client will

A. have a slight loss of hearing pattern

B. demonstrate pain control at a level of 5

C. experience a small loss of auditory perception

D. demonstrate an understanding of the condition and medication regimen

5. The nurse identifies which of the following as a component of the middle ear?

A. lobule

B. pinna

C. eustachian tube

D. cochlea

6. The nurse instructs the client that the best way to prevent cerumen impaction is to

A. instill 3 cc of half-strength hydrogen peroxide in the ear at bedtime

B. never use cotton swabs in the ear canal

C. allow water from the shower to run into the ear canal when taking a shower

D. irrigate the ear with benzocaine

7. A new nurse is administering a wax emulsifier to an adult client. Which action by the nurse requires the supervising nurse to intervene? The new nurse

A. pulls the pinna up

B. pulls the pinna outward

C. pulls the pinna down

D. uses clean procedure

8. Which statement by a client indicates that more teaching about use of otic medications is indicated?

A. "I will store the medication in the refrigerator."

B. "I will avoid use of cotton-tipped applicators in my ears."

C. "I will take the medication as prescribed."

D. "I will tilt my head to the opposite side of where the ear medication will been instilled."

9. While waiting for the effect of an anesthetic or analgesic medication for the ear to take effect, the nurse should have the client

A. lie on the affected ear

B. place ice on the affected ear

C. instill a moisturizer into the ear canal of the affected ear

D. Place a warm, clean cloth over the affected ear

10. Which of the following statements about otitis media does the nurse identify as true?

A. It is the most common inner ear infection.

B. It usually occurs after an individual has a gastrointestinal infection.

C. It is the leading cause of conductive hearing loss in children.

D. It only occurs in children.

Multiple Response

Circle the best answers for each of the following questions. More than one answer is correct.

1. Which of the following statements about conditions of the ear will the nurse include in client teaching? Select all that apply.

A. Otitis media is the most common middle ear disorder.

B. Otitis media occurs in children.

C. Otitis media occurs in adults.

D. Dental caries can cause otitis media.

E. Otitis media most often results in sensioneural hearing loss.

F. It is most often caused by a fungal infection.

2. Which of the following will the nurse include when teaching a client about wax emulsifiers? Select all that apply.
   A. Hearing loss can result from impacted cerumen.
   B. Bacterial growth can result from impacted cerumen.
   C. The best way to prevent cerumen impaction is to clean the ear canal daily with cotton swabs.
   D. Impacted cerumen is best removed by using a thin plastic tube to break up the impacted wax.
   E. Wax emulsifiers should be administered at room temperature.
   F. Over-the-counter wax emulsifiers are most often used twice daily.

Critical Thinking Exercises

1. Develop a teaching plan focused on the prevention of the development of otitis media in children as well as adults.

   _____

   _____

   _____

   _____

2. Create a care plan for your client with an otitis media infection, including nursing interventions. Specify techniques for promoting pain relief and positive well-being.

   _____

   _____

   _____

   _____

3. Using Microsoft PowerPoint, create a presentation to illustrate how an infant's or child's ear anatomy differs from that of an adult.

   _____

   _____

   _____

   _____

CHAPTER 42 *Agents Used in the Treatment of Skin Conditions*

Objectives

After reading Chapter 42 of *Pharmacological Aspects of Nursing Care,* 8th edition, the student will be able to:

1. Discuss the properties of and specific uses for ointments, creams, pastes, lotions, gels, aerosol sprays, aerosol foams, powders, oils, and tapes when used in the treatment of dermatological disorders.
2. Discuss five causes of dry skin.
3. Explain the role of emollients in relieving dry skin.
4. Describe the therapeutic use and appropriate method of application of topical skin agents.
5. Discuss adverse effects, drug interactions, and contraindications related to the use of topical agents on the skin.
6. Discuss the appropriate use of antimicrobial agents in the treatment of topical skin infections.
7. Discuss the factors to be assessed in clients receiving treatment for skin disorders.
8. Describe in a stepwise manner the procedure used in the application of a cream or ointment.
9. Apply the nursing process related to the administration of agents used in the treatment of dermatological disorders.
10. Apply the nursing process for clients being treated for burns.
11. Successfully complete the games and activities in the online student StudyWARE.

Definitions

Supply the definitions for the following terms.

1. emollient _____
2. keratolytic agent _____
3. antipruritic _____
4. sebaceous glands _____
5. stratum germinativum _____
6. antiviral agent _____
7. apocrine glands _____
8. actinic ketatoses _____

Fill in the Blank

Write in the missing information.

1. Treatment of dry skin is often best accomplished by the use of _____.
2. Skin disorders such as _____, _____, _____, _____, _____, and _____ are characterized by thickening of the keratin layer of the skin.
3. Local anesthetic agents can be used in the treatment of clients with skin conditions to reduce _____ and _____.
4. Dermatophyte infections are usually caused by _____ and similar organisms.
5. Most dermatological yeast infections are caused by _____.

Multiple Choice

Circle the best answer for each of the following questions. There is only one answer to each question.

1. Grafts from the client's own skin are called

   A. autografts
   B. allografts
   C. xenografts
   D. heterografts

2. A new nurse is using an emollient on a client. The supervising nurse should intervene if the new nurse

   A. applies the emollient after bathing the client
   B. applies the emollient to exudative skin
   C. limits the application to the area of skin in need of treatment
   D. applies the emollient after the client has taken a shower

3. Which statement by a client using a keratolytic agent indicates that more education is needed?

   A. "I will apply the agent after I take a shower."
   B. "I will apply a dressing over the keratolytic."
   C. "I will apply the keratolytic at night and remove it in the morning."
   D. "I will take a pain medication before applying the keratolytic agent."

4. Which of the following dermatologic agents does the nurse identify as being best able to absorb secretions from skin lesions?

   A. ointment
   B. cream
   C. paste
   D. lotion

5. Which of the following items does the nurse identify as most effective in the treatment of a client with excess friction between body parts?

   A. powder
   B. oil
   C. tape
   D. bead

6. Which of the following statements about yeast infections of the skin does the nurse identify as being true?

   A. Moisture retards yeast growth.
   B. Antifungal products should be applied once daily.
   C. The antifungal product should be applied for 1 week after disappearance of lesions.
   D. Topical therapy of yeast infections is generally successful within 10 days of therapy.

7. When working with a client who has sustained a burn injury, it is most important for the nurse to assess the client for the development of

   A. edema
   B. infection
   C. electrolyte disturbances
   D. cardiac dysrhythmias

8. Use of which of the following medications often result in dark red colored urine?

   A. silver sulfadiazine
   B. mafenide
   C. nitrofurazone
   D. minoxidil

9. A client is taking minoxidil. It is most important for the nurse to assess the client for a history of

   A. diabetes mellitus
   B. heart disease
   C. chronic obstructive pulmonary disease
   D. renal impairment

10. When working with a client who is receiving treatment for a burn injury, the nurse will

    A. medicate the client for pain after the dressing change
    B. assess the patient receiving silver nitrate for the development of metabolic acidosis
    C. cleanse the wound from the outside to the center
    D. keep silver nitrate dressings wet to avoid the solution becoming caustic to tissues

Multiple Response

Circle the best answers for each of the following questions. More than one answer is correct.

1. The nurse identifies which of the following as functions of the skin? Select all that apply.

   A. prevention of loss of protein from the body
   B. prevention of microbiological intruders
   C. thermoregulation
   D. excretory organ
   E. manufacturing of vitamin C
   F. site of bone manufacturing

2. Which of the following does the nurse identify as a localized allergic reaction to the administration of local anesthetics to the skin? Select all that apply.

   A. cyanosis
   B. erythema
   C. urticaria
   D. edema
   E. alopecia
   F. jaundice

Critical Thinking Exercises

1. Visit a local store that sells products for treatment of disorders of the skin. Share findings with the class. How many different products were identified?

   _____

   _____

   _____

   _____

2. When in the clinical area, identify the types of products used to treat dermatologic conditions as well as products to prevent the development of alterations in skin integrity.

   _____

   _____

   _____

   _____

3. Compare and contrast nursing responsibilities associated with antimicrobial agents used to treat dermatologic conditions.

   _____

   _____

   _____

   _____

4. Develop a plan of care for the client receiving treatment for psoriasis and eczema.

_____

_____

_____

_____

5. Develop a plan of care for a client who has sustained a burn injury specific to topical drug therapy.

_____

_____

_____

_____

ANSWER KEY

Chapter 1

Definitions
1. the study of absorption, distribution, metabolism, and excretion of drugs
2. the study of how drugs are used in the treatment of illness
3. the study of how a person responds to a drug
4. the study of drugs derived from herbs
5. the study of a drug's mechanism of action

Fill in the Blank
1. Toxicology
2. tablet
3. Syrups
4. Emulsions
5. synergistically

Multiple Choice
1. A   6. C
2. B   7. A
3. D   8. B
4. C   9. C
5. C   10. A

Multiple Response
1. C, D, E
2. A, B, D, E

Chapter 2

Definitions
1. within the cavity of a joint
2. into the spinal fluid
3. also called vaginal irrigations, occasionally prescribed to promote comfort and remove secretions
4. into the dermis of the skin
5. administration of a drug by a route other than the intestinal tract

Fill in the Blank
1. right drug, right dose, right client, right time, right route, right documentation, client's right to refuse
2. 20–30 minutes
3. at eye level
4. 90
5. up and back

Multiple Choice

1. C	6. A
2. B	7. C
3. D	8. A
4. D	9. D
5. B	10. B

Multiple Response

1. E, F
2. B, D, E, F

Chapter 3

Definitions

1. the force water exerts against vessel walls
2. the amount of hydrostatic pressure needed to move particles and fluids in and out of vascular volume
3. solutions that raise oncotic pressure
4. solutions that do not alter plasma osmolality
5. solutions that create osmotic pressure by dissolved ion movement

Fill in the Blank

1. maintaining the patency of the intravenous access
2. Venipuncture
3. Thrombophlebitis
4. extravasation
5. pyrogenic reaction

Multiple Choice

1. B	6. B
2. A	7. D
3. D	8. C
4. C	9. A
5. C	10. A

Multiple Response

1. D, E, F
2. B, D, E, F

Chapter 4

Definitions

1. the relationship of two quantities
2. formed by using two equal ratios
3. the basic unit of weight in the metric system
4. the basic unit of volume in the metric system

Fill in the Blank

1. left
2. right
3. grams
4. milligrams per kilogram
5. nomogram

Practice Problems

1. 0.5 mL
2. 1 tablet
3. 1.25 mL
4. 8 mL
5. 250 mL
6. 4 capsules
7. ½ tablet
8. 2 tablets
9. 12 mL
10. 10 mg; 5 mg/dose
11. ½ mL
12. 50 gtt/min
13. 12.5 mL/hour
14. 8 hours
15. 200 mL/hour

Chapter 5

Definitions

1. a substance previously routinely used to induce vomiting in the treatment of vomiting
2. agents used by health care professionals to prevent gastric absorption of poisons
3. a herb known to contain powerful diuretic compounds

Fill in the Blank

1. sparingly
2. Renal
3. Electronic infusion devices

Multiple Choice

1. A
2. B
3. C
4. B
5. D
6. D
7. D
8. A
9. D
10. B

Multiple Response

1. A, E, F
2. A, B

Chapter 6

Definitions

1. the metabolism of a drug
2. a test used to determine renal function
3. a disease of the heart that results in reduced cardiac output and reduced gastrointestional blood flow resulting in reduced absorption of drugs

Fill in the Blank
1. reduction
2. decline
3. renal function

Multiple Choice
1. B
2. A
3. A
4. B
5. D

6. A
7. B
8. C
9. D
10. D

Multiple Response
1. A, C, F
2. B, C, D

Chapter 7

Definitions
1. the person or animal that becomes infected with the infectious agent
2. the process by which the infectious agent is passed on: blood, body fluids, feces, food, water, fecal-oral contamination
3. the person or animal that carries the infectious agent; this person or animal may not be infected themselves
4. the process by which the microorganism is removed from the reservoir: through blood, feces, droplets, or body fluids
5. the process by which the microorganism gains entry into the fomite or vector
6. the disease-causing microorganism responsible for starting the infectious process
7. agents that either destroy or inhibit the growth of both pathogenic and nonpathogenic bacteria
8. agents that inhibit the growth of bacteria
9. agents useful in treating infections in which the identify and susceptibility to antimicrobial treatment of the infecting organism(s) has not been established
10. agents that have a killing action on the microbial agent
11. among the simplest living organisms, they are able to enter living cells to sustain their growth and reproduce
12. a rapid method for establishing the biochemical nature of the bacterial cell wall, either gram-positive or gram-negative; on the basis of this information, an antimicrobial agent effective in eradicating the organism can be chosen

Fill in the Blank
1. age, exposure to pathogenic organisms, disruption of the body's normal barriers to infection, inadequate immunological defenses, impaired circulation, and poor nutritional status
2. Bactericidal; bacteriostatic
3. Viruses
4. rash, urticaria, fever, bronchospasm, in extreme cases, anaphylaxis
5. penicillins
6. cephalosporins
7. tetracyclines
8. macrolides
9. Psdueomonas aeruginosa
10. HIV infection

11. doxycycline; tetracycline

12. leprosy

Multiple Choice

1. A
2. A
3. D
4. B
5. C
6. D
7. C
8. B
9. C
10. C
11. E

Multiple Response

1. C, D, F
2. A, B, D, E
3. D, E, F

Chapter 8

Definitions

1. one of the safest and most effective antimalarials currently available
2. infestation of parasitic worms
3. parasitic disease characterized by invasion of the large bowel by protozoa
4. protozoa infection characterized by recurrent chills, fever, and prostration
5. may be contracted by person-to-person contact, insects, direct contact with parasites or bed linens, or contaminated food or water
6. the most useful drug in the treatment of amebiasis

Fill in the Blank

1. dermatologic, gastrointestinal, or systemic
2. Plasmodium
3. bite of a mosquito; transfusions of blood that contain the organism; injections with syringes or needles that have been used by an affected individual
4. Entamoeba histolytica
5. rheumatoid arthritis; discoid lupus erythematosus
6. Metronidazole
7. Helminthiasis, or infestation with parasitic worms,
8. darken; reddish brown

Multiple Choice

1. A
2. A
3. C
4. A
5. A
6. A
7. C
8. C
9. A
10. C

Multiple Response

1. A, B, E, F
2. C, D

Chapter 9

Definitions

1. destroys pathogenic microorganisms and helps to prevent infection
2. kills or inhibits growth of microorganisms
3. capable of destroying microorganisms
4. preventative
5. inhibits itching
6. liberation of oxygen gas when hydrogen peroxide rapidly breaks down after exposure to catalse found in living tissue
7. seal off flow

Fill in the Blank

1. Cresol (Lysol)
2. Formaldehyde
3. phenol
4. Silver nitrate
5. triclocarban
6. isopropyl alcohol (isopropanol)
7. Thimerosal (Mersol)
8. Hand hygiene

Multiple Choice

1. D	6. A
2. A	7. D
3. C	8. A
4. C	9. D
5. A	10. B

Multiple Response

1. A, B
2. A, B, C, F

Chapter 10

Definitions

1. the level of stimulus resulting in the perception of pain
2. relieves pain without causing a loss of consciousness
3. the amount of pain an individual can withstand without disrupting normal functions or requiring analgesic therapy
4. endogenous analgesic compounds that are released when painful stimuli affect the body
5. a sense of detachment and well-being
6. a physiological response to the removal of a drug from the body characterized by the development of signs and symptoms such as sweating, restlessness, and diarrhea, which are often related to the body's overcompensation to the discontinuation of the drug
7. "Pain is what the client says it is."
8. the self-administration of intravenous doses of opioid analgesics using a special infusion pump

Fill in the Blank

1. gate theory of pain
2. endorphins; enkephalins
3. Morphine sulfate
4. morphine sulfate
5. morphine sulfate
6. Rylomine

Multiple Choice

1. A
2. B
3. B
4. D
5. A

6. B
7. D
8. A
9. C
10. D

Multiple Response

1. A, C, F
2. A, B, C, F
3. C, D, E, F

Chapter 11

Definitions

1. Provides sedation and relieves pre-op anxiety but does not depress respirations.
2. Agents that interfere with nerve conduction and cause diminished pain and sensation.
3. Partial or complete loss of consciousness.
4. Blocks nerves only in a specific area and does not cause loss of consciousness.
5. Anesthetic is injected into the subarachnoid or epidural space surrounding the spinal cord.
6. An unexpected fever occurring while the client is anesthetized and possibly when exposed to intensive exercise and certain other stressors.

Fill in the Blank

1. nerve conduction
2. Regional anesthetics
3. analgesia, excitement or delirium,surgical anesthesia, medullary paralysis
4. General anesthesia
5. diminish salivation, prevent laryngospasm, prevent reflex bradycardia
6. cocaine
7. Dantrolene (Dantrium)
8. 6–12

Multiple Choice

1. B
2. D
3. A
4. A
5. C
6. B

7. D
8. A
9. B
10. C
11. D
12. B

Multiple Response
1. D, F
2. A, B, C, D, E
3. B, C, D, E, F

Chapter 12

Definition
1. vascular and delayed cellular response to invaders or injury
2. group of synthetic medications that work by inhibiting prostaglandins
3. group of drugs that dramatically reduce inflammation but have negative effect of suppressing the body's immune response
4. newest of the DMARDs act by inhibiting steps of the inflammatory process associated with RA
5. group of drugs used for the treatment of inflammation
6. substances made in the adrenal cortex that act on the distal tubules of the kidney
7. most potent prostaglandin inhibitor and anti-inflammatory agent
8. important mediators in the inflammatory process
9. substance secreted by the adrenal cortex
10. type of NSAID that provides anti-inflammatory action with much lower gastrointestinal effects and no effects on platelet aggregation

Fill in the Blank
1. thrombotic event, MI, CVA, hypertension
2. aspirin
3. serious infection and increased risk of malignancies
4. herpes zoster or shingles
5. retinal damage

Multiple Choice

1. C	6. C
2. D	7. B
3. A	8. A
4. D	9. C
5. B	10. B

Multiple Response
1. A, D, F
2. B, C, F

Chapter 13

Definitions
1. a metabolic disease caused by hyperuricemia
2. presence of abnormally elevated amounts of uric acid in the blood
3. crystals deposits in tissues and joints from body fluids saturated with uric acid precipitates
4. a condition characterized by inflammation at the site of crystal deposition and acute joint pain
5. an agent such as probenicid whicy that acts to increase the urinary excretion of uric acid

Fill in the Blank

1. low dose aspirin therapy, thiazide diuretics, immunosuppressant drugs such as cyclosporin used in transplantation

2. African American men

3. protein

4. metatarsophalangeal

5. high doses of nonsteroidal anti-inflammatory drugs

Multiple Choice

1. B
2. B
3. A
4. C
5. B
6. B
7. D
8. A
9. C
10. A

Multiple Response

1. A, D, E
2. A, D, E

Chapter 14

Definitions

1. a naturally occurring substance in the body released in response to tissue damage and the presence of microorganisms and allergens invading body tissue

2. excess fluid due to the use of topical decongestants when used longer than recommended

3. a medication used to relieve coughing

4. a process by which an individual is slowly and safely exposed to an offending allergen

5. the antihistamine Allegra

Fill in the Blank

1. The common cold, allergic rhinitis

2. a viral infection

3. pharyngitis

4. histamine

5. inhibit lactation

6. Diphenhydramine (Bendadryl)

7. alpha 1-adrenergic

8. hypertension, glaucoma, prostate problems

Multiple Choice

1. C
2. A
3. C
4. D
5. C
6. C
7. A
8. C
9. B
10. B

Multiple Response

1. A, B, C
2. C, D, E, F

Chapter 15

Definitions
1. a collection of respiratory diseases that impairs respiratory function
2. first leukotriene receptor antagonist used for the treatment of asthma
3. natural surfactant derived from the lungs of cows
4. unrelieved asthma attack lasting for an extended period of time; may be fatal
5. most commonly used mucolytic agent
6. mast cell stabilizer most commonly used for the prophylactic treatment of bronchial asthma in clients who require long-term therapy to control their disease and whose attacks follow a predictable pattern
7. first drug therapy approved by the FDA to treat allergy-related asthma
8. agents that reduce thickness and stickiness of pulmonary secretions so removal by ciliary action and cough is facilitated and pulmonary ventilation can be improved

Fill in the Blank
1. airway edema, smooth muscle construction, altered cellular activity
2. copper, rubber, iron
3. 10–20 mcg/mL
4. monoamine oxidase inhibitors (MAOs)
5. zafirlukust (Accolate), montelukast (Singulair)
6. tachycardia, cardiac arrhythmia, gastrointestinal symptoms

Multiple Choice
1. C
2. B
3. B
4. D
5. A
6. B
7. C
8. D
9. A
10. C

Multiple Response
1. A, B, E, F
2. A, C, E, F

Chapter 16

Definitions
1. a cardiac glycoside that decreases the velocity of electrical conduction and prolongs the refractory period in the atrioventricular conduction system of the heart
2. increases the force of the heart's contractions
3. reduces the force of the heart's contractions
4. increases the heart rate by altering the rate of impulse formation at the sinoatrial (SA) node
5. a decrease in the rate of electrical conduction
6. an increase in the rate of electrical conduction
7. drugs that work by decreasing automaticity, altering conduction rates, or altering the refractory period between cardiac contractions

8. the structure that generates an electrical impulse in the heart located between the atria and ventricles

9. the pacemaker of the heart

10. the ability of the heart to spontaneously initiate electrical activity

Fill in the Blank

1. sodium potassium ATPase

2. myosin

3. Digoxin

4. 0.5–2.0

5. Vaughan-Williams

6. Lidocaine

7. Phenytoin (Dilantin)

8. angina

9. antacids

10. pulmonary toxicity

Multiple Choice

1. C
2. D
3. C
4. C
5. A
6. A
7. A
8. D
9. C
10. D
11. B
12. D

Multiple Response

1. B, C, D, E, F

2. C, E, F

Chapter 17

Definitions

1. a consequence of the dilation of cerebral blood vessels when nitrate therapy is used

2. a beta-adrenergic blocker used in the treatment of angina pectoris

3. area of the heart muscle dies as a result of insufficient oxygen

4. a calcium-channel blocker used in the treatment of angina pectoris

5. a nitrate used in the treatment of angina

Fill in the Blank

1. Nitroglycerine

2. obstructive pulmonary disease, asthma, congestive heart failure, greater than first degree heart block, bradycardia, diabetes melllitus

3. hypotensive episodes

4. 325 mg aspirin, intravenous morphine sulfate

5. 6

6. 5% dextrose injection, 0.9% sodium chloride injection

Multiple Choice

1.	A	6.	D
2.	A	7.	B
3.	C	8.	B
4.	A	9.	A
5.	B	10.	B

Multiple Response

1. B, C, E
2. A, B, C, F
3. A, C, F

Chapter 18

Definitions

1. safest diuretic agents currently in use; appear to act by inhibiting sodium and chloride reabsorption in the early portion of the distal tubule; may result in hypokalemia

2. agents that cause a high concentration of osmotic agents in the kidney tubule, which leads to large amounts of fluid and produces a profound diuretic effect

3. an abnormal increase in arterial blood pressure; normal blood pressure is defined as less than 120 mmHg systolic and less than 80mmHg diastolic

4. drugs that interfere with the conversion of angiotensin I to angiotensin II by inhibiting the action of ACE, resulting in dilation of peripheral blood vessels and a reduction in blood pressure

5. agents used to reduce arterial blood pressure at rest and during exercise by dilating peripheral arterioles and reducing peripheral resistance

Fill in the Blank

1. potassium, chloride
2. hearing loss
3. less than 120 mmHg, less than 80 mmHg
4. Diet Approach, Stop Hypertension
5. nitroprusside, fenoldopam, labetolol HCl

Multiple Choice

1.	C	6.	D
2.	D	7.	A
3.	A	8.	B
4.	A	9.	D
5.	C	10.	B

Multiple Response

1. D, E, F
2. C, D, E, F

Chapter 19

Definitions
1. excessive buildup of cholesterol and plaque on blood vessel walls
2. the smallest lipoprotein with the highest proportion of protein
3. substances that contain the greatest proportion of cholesterol of all lipoproteins
4. substances secreted in the liver that have a triglyceride component partially derived from dietary carbohydrate intake
5. a type of lipoprotein that contains the highest proportion of lipid and is therefore the least dense of the lipoprotein particles
6. class of drugs that inhibit the action of the enzyme HMG-CoA reductase, resulting in an increase in HDL cholesterol and a reduction of triglyceride levels

Fill in the Blank
1. very low-density lipoproteins (VLDL), low-density lipoproteins (LDL)
2. HMG-CoA reductase inhibitors
3. 200, 100, 150, 40
4. Rhabdomyolysis
5. limitation of dietary fat and cholesterol, weight reduction, regular exercise

Multiple Choice

1. C	6. C
2. A	7. D
3. C	8. D
4. D	9. A
5. C	10. B

Multiple Response
1. A, C
2. A, B, D, E, F

Chapter 20

Definitions
1. substances that inhibit the action or formation of one or more clotting factors
2. an agent found in mast cells that is a potent inhibitor of the clotting process
3. lack of prothrombine often caused by an overdose of anticoagulants
4. synthetic analog of the posterior pituitary hormone shown to increase Factor VIII levels within 30 minutes after administration by the IV route
5. a blood clot
6. agents used to stop the flow of blood in cases of excessive bleeding

Fill in the Blank
1. bioassay
2. a slow infusion of 1% protamine sulfate solution
3. antihistamines, digitalis, ginsing, goldenrod, nicotine,nitroglycerine, tetracyclines
4. 12–24
5. p\Prothrombin time, INR

6. 1.5–2.5
7. prothrombin
8. orally
9. subcutaneously, intravenously
10. Abciximab (ReoPro)

Multiple Choice

1. B	7. B
2. A	8. C
3. C	9. A
4. A	10. C
5. D	11. B
6. D	12. A

Multiple Response

1. A, B, C, F
2. C, D, E
3. C, F

Chapter 21

Definitions

1. a relatively uncommon genetic disease in which antibodies are formed against intrinsic factor
2. common form of anemia usually caused by blood loss or a dietary deficiency of iron
3. a substance secreted by the kidney that acts to stimulate red blood cell production
4. a synthetic form of Vitamin B_{12} used for parenteral therapy
5. an ESA administered subcutaneously used for the treatment of anemia in clients with cancer

Fill in the Blank

1. ferrous sulfate
2. uncontrolled hypertension
3. weakness, sore tongue, numbing or tingling of the extremities
4. folic acid
5. deferoxamine mesylate

Multiple Choice

1. C	6. A
2. B	7. C
3. A	8. D
4. C	9. A
5. B	10. B

Multiple Response

1. D, E, F
2. A, C, F

Chapter 22

Definitions
1. substances needed for chemical reactions, maintenance of health, and growth
2. divided into two groups: major elements and micro elements
3. vitamins A, D, E, and K; stored by the body
4. thiamine, folic acid and vitamin C are dissolved in water, eliminated in urine, and are not stored by the body thus requiring a continuous supply in our diets
5. proteins and fat bound together to facilitate transport
6. this nutrient is 4 kcal/g and is used for the synthesis, maintenance, and repair of body tissues
7. sugars and starches
8. concentrated source of fatty acids, 9 kcal/g
9. serum sodium concentration is greater than 145 mEq/L
10. proteins, carbohydrates, and fats

Fill in the Blank
1. vitamins, minerals
2. C
3. 8
4. Vitamin K
5. thiamine
6. folic acid
7. cardiac arrhythmias
8. tetany

Multiple Choice
1. A
2. B
3. C
4. B
5. C
6. A
7. D
8. A
9. A
10. D
11. A
12. B

Multiple Response
1. B, C, E, F
2. A, B, C, D

Chapter 23

Definitions
1. overproduction of hydrochloric acid
2. bacterium known to invade the gastrointestinal lining causing peptic ulcer disease
3. a synthetic prostaglandin compound reported to decrease gastric acid secretion and possibly exert a protective effect on the mucosal surface of the stomach
4. a chemical derivative of sucrose that adheres to the ulcer and protects it from further acid attack
5. a drug that stimulates the motility of the upper gastrointestinal tract without stimulating the production of gastric, biliary, or pancreatic secretions

Fill in the Blank

1. Simethicone

2. antiadrogenic, central nervous system

3. Esomeprazole magnesium

4. Misoprostol

5. yogurt, hard cheese

Multiple Choice

1. C	6. B
2. A	7. D
3. C	8. A
4. C	9. B
5. D	10. A

Multiple Response

1. D, F

2. B, C, D

Chapter 24

Definitions

1. agents that block serotonin receptors in the gastrointestinal tract that cause nausea and vomiting

2. agents used to prevent and treat nausea and vomiting

3. also known as dopamine antagonists, agents that act by binding with dopamine$_2$ receptors to minimize the effect of dopamine and to limit emetic input in the medullary emetic center

4. agents that block dopamine and stimulate acetylcholine to increase gastric emptying

5. antiemetic agent commonly used to treat postoperative nausea associated with general anesthesia

6. a 5-HT3 receptor antagonist used to treat nausea and vomiting associated with chemotherapy

Fill in the Blank

1. dry mouth, urinary retention, blurred vision

2. orthostatic hypotension, sedation, tardive dyskinesia

3. ondansetron

4. diphenhydramine

5. 1 hour

Multiple Choice

1. B	6. C
2. B	7. A
3. D	8. C
4. D	9. D
5. D	10. A

Multiple Response

1. D, E, F

2. A, C, D, E

Chapter 25

Definitions
1. agents used to permit easier mixing of fat and fluids in the fecal mass
2. agents that absorb fluid in the intestine, causing swelling of the intestine and promoting peristalsis
3. condition in which the passage of feces is slow or nonexistent
4. synthetic disaccharide containing the monosaccharides galactose and fructose; the sugar is not digested and passes to the colon unchanged producing a laxative effect
5. laxatives that facilitate the passage of fecal mass through the intestine by maintaining hydration of the fecal mass
6. abnormal frequent passage of watery stool
7. class of medications used to reduce gastrointestinal motility
8. condition in which the client requires larger and larger doses of an agent for appropriate defecation

Fill in the Blank
1. stimulant laxatives
2. Hyperosmolar laxatives
3. milk
4. oils
5. opium derivatives, anticholinergic agents

Multiple Choice
1. D
2. A
3. B
4. B
5. B
6. C
7. B
8. A
9. B
10. D

Multiple Response
1. A, B, C
2. A, B, D, E

Chapter 26

Definitions
1. also referred to as anxiolytics, these agents reduce nervousness and anxiety without causing sleep *sedatives*
2. central nervous system depressants that potentiate gamma-aminobutyric acid (GABA) mediated neural inhibition *Benzo*
3. agents that produce central nervous system depression and anticonvulsant activity *barb*
4. agents that cause relaxation and promote sleep *hypnotics*
5. also called alcohol; fairly potent central nervous system depressant *ethenol*

Fill in the Blank
1. Benzodiazepines
2. Flumazenil
3. kava rhizone, valerian root
4. asthma, glaucoma
5. anticonvulsant

Multiple Choice

1.	C	6.	C
2.	A	7.	D
3.	D	8.	A
4.	B	9.	B
5.	D		

Multiple Response
1. A, D, E
2. A, B, C, F

Chapter 27

Definitions
1. agents used to treat emotional and psychiatric conditions *psychotropic drugs*
2. suggests that alterations in neurotransmitters in the central nervous system are responsible for the depressed state
3. agents that suppress spontaneous movement and complex behaviors but do not alter spinal reflexes *neuroleptics*
4. changes of mood *affective disorders*
5. extrapyramidal symptoms (EPS) that usuallly appear after 2 or more years of antipsychotic drug therapy *dyskinesia*
6. agents used to treat anxiety disorders *anxiolytics*
7. also known as MAOs, agents commonly used in the treatment of depression *MOI*
8. neurotransmitter responsible for mood *serotonin*

Fill in the Blank
1. barbiturates, antihistamines, carbamates, benzodiazepines
2. Doxepin HCl
3. selective serotonin reuptake inhibitors (SSRIs)
4. 2–3 weeks
5. chlorpromazine (Thorazine)
6. Akathisia
7. Tardive dyskinesia
8. Antipsychotic

Multiple Choice

1.	B	5.	A
2.	C	6.	B
3.	D	7.	A
4.	D	8.	C

Multiple Response
1. A, B, C, D
2. A, C, E, F

Chapter 28

Definitions

1. drug used in the treatment of Alzheimer's disease that inhibits cholinesterase, thereby increasing acetycholine in the cerebral cortex *tacrine*

2. neurobehavioral disorder characterized by hyperkinetic-impulsive or inattentive manifestations that cause impairment and are present before the age of 7 years *ADHD*

3. progressive, degenerative, terminal disease of the brain tissue that is the leading cause of dementia *Alzheimer*

4. agents used for the treatment of respiratory depression caused by narcotics or other central nervous system depressants *analeptics*

5. also known as anorexiants, these agents depress the appetite *anoretic agents*

6. a N-methylD-aspartate antagonist used in the treatment of Alzheimer's disease that acts to alter levels of acetylcholine *memantine*

7. a CNS stimulant that stimulates the medullary center of the brain to increase depth of respiration; ABG's must be monitored carefully before starting this therapy *doxapram*

8. condition characterized by attacks of sleep occurring throughout the day *narcolepsy*

Fill in the Blank

1. neurofibrillary tangles, senile plaques
2. Caffeine
3. inattention, hyperactivity, impulsivity
4. Caffeine
5. IV atropine sulfate

Multiple Choice

1. C	6. B
2. A	7. C
3. A	8. C
4. A	9. D
5. C	10. C

Multiple Response

1. A, C, E
2. B, D, F

Chapter 29

Definitions

1. intentional paralysis using medications that paralyze skeletal muscle groups, but do not affect cardiac muscle

2. agents that relax skeletal muscle by their action on the CNS that are used in the treatment of clients with acute muscle spasm associated with sprains, strains, and other acute traumatic conditions involving skeletal muscles

3. test used in the diagnosis of myasthenia gravis that is positive in 75% of clients with myasthenia gravis

4. response to overmedication with anticholinesterase drugs; manifestations include lacrimation, salivation, diarrhea, intestinal cramping, bradycardia and miosis

5. anticholinesterase drug used in the treatment of clients with myasthenia gravis that has long duration of action

Fill in the Blank
1. pyridostigmine, edrophonium
2. Dantrolene
3. Myasthenia gravis
4. Ropinirole HCl
5. Pyridostigmine bromide

Multiple Choice

1. C
2. C
3. D
4. A
5. A
6. C
7. A
8. C
9. A
10. D

Multiple Response
1. A, B, C
2. B, C, D, E

Chapter 30

Definitions
1. (Sinemet) used in the treatment of PD to prevent levodopa breakdown in the peripheral circulation, allowing more levodopa to be available for entry into the brain and less dopamine stored in the peripheral circulation thereby substantially reducing the incidence of severity of drug-related adverse effects
2. anti-Parkinson agent that acts by releasing dopamine from central neurons, thereby increasing dopamine concentrations in the CNS
3. drug used to treat clients with a "frozen" undermedicated state of PD; must be administered SQ, acts within 4-8 minutes with the period of improvement lasting 45–60 minutes; for short-term management only
4. agents used to treat PD that act by reducing excessive cholinergic activity in the brain
5. drug used to treat PD that may cause urine to darken

Fill in the Blank
1. muscle tremor, rigidity, lack of coordination
2. acetylcholine, dopamine
3. palliative
4. malignant melanoma
5. vitamin B_6, protein

Multiple Choice

1. C
2. B
3. D
4. D
5. C
6. C
7. C
8. B
9. A
10. C

Multiple Response
1. B, E, F
2. D, E, F

Chapter 31

Definitions

1. an anticonvulsant medication used to treat certain partial seizures in adults and as an adjunct in the treatment of seizures associated with Lennox-Gastaunt syndrome in children

2. an anticonvulsant that has shown the best results in treating absence seizures in children

3. anticonvulsant drug also found to be effective in the treatment of trigeminal neuralgia

4. formerly called petit mal seizures, they are characterized by staring and occasional fluttering of the eyes that begins and ends abruptly

5. formerly called grand mal seizures, these seizures involve both hemispheres of the brain at onset and are characterized by a sudden cry, falling, and rigidity followed by muscle jerks, shallow breathing, or temporary apnea, and possible loss of bowel and bladder control

6. a benzodiazepine administered intravenously as the drug of choice for treating status epilepticus

7. clusters of jerking movements exhibited by children between the ages of 3 months and 2 years

8. a series of tonic-clonic seizures without a return of consciousness between seizures

9. seizures that do not respond to traditional pharmacologic anticonvulsant therapy

10. antiepileptic drugs

Fill in the Blank

1. central nervous system
2. diazepam
3. sodium
4. sulfonamides
5. intramuscular

Multiple Choice

1. C	6. D
2. A	7. A
3. C	8. A
4. B	9. A
5. B	10. D

Multiple Response

1. A, B, D
2. A, E, F

Chapter 32

Definitions

1. overwhelming compulsion to participate in unhealthy behavior despite negative consequences

2. intense cravings (but not physical discomfort) cause a person to use a substance

3. biological condition where the body adapts to a substance and its repeated administration

4. central nervous system (CNS) adapts to repeated substance use and suffers withdrawal symptoms if the substance is not used

5. once tolerance develops to a certain substance, the tolerance extends to chemically related drugs

6. drug whose primary action is to alter perception and cognition; part of a class of drugs known as hallucinogens

Fill in the Blank

1. Habituation

2. Tolerance

3. buprenophine, methadone

4. Alcohol (ethanol)

5. higher

6. carbon monoxide, nicotine, tars, smoke particles

Multiple Choice

1. A	6. C
2. C	7. B
3. B	8. D
4. A	9. C
5. D	10. A

Multiple Response

1. A, B, E, F

2. A, B, F

Chapter 33

Definitions

1. chemical messengers that transmit impulses

2. the cholinergic branch of the autonomic nervous system (ANS)

3. a single-neuron system

4. the adrenergic branch of the autonomic nervous system

5. cluster of nerve cell bodies

6. located primarily in the smooth muscle of peripheral blood vessels, urinary, and gastrointestinal sphincters

7. located on the presynaptic neuron

8. block or inhibit the responses of adrenergic neurotransmitters

9. found in the smooth muscle of the heart and in fatty tissue

10. located primarily in bronchial smooth muscles and in blood vessels in the heart, brain, and skeletal muscle

11. the sympathetic (adrenergic) branch of the autonomic nervous system

12. located in brown adipose tissue, they regulate thermogenesis and lipolysis when stimulated by norepinephrine

Fill in the Blank

1. parasympathetic

2. parasympathetic, sympathetic

3. catecholamines

4. decrease

5. dilate (mydriasis)

6. acetylcholine

7. Dicyclomine HCl

8. emesis, aspiration

9. pyridostigmine, edrophonium, neostigmine

10. dilate

Multiple Choice

1. A	6. A
2. D	7. A
3. D	8. B
4. A	9. B
5. D	10. B

Multiple Response

1. B, D, F
2. B, C, E, F

Chapter 34

Definitions

1. excessive secretion of thyroid hormone by the thyroid gland resulting in increased levels of metabolism in virtually all physiological systems within the body
2. state of the thyroid when agents have been used to suppress its function
3. thyroid hormone deficiency that can be caused by a number of different disease states
4. pinhead-sized structures located behind the thyroid gland whose primary function is the secretion of parathyroid hormone in response to a reduction of the serum calcium level
5. deficiency of parathyroid hormone that results in low serum calcium levels, elevated phosphorus levels, and a wide array of symptoms including increased neuromuscular irritability and psychiatric disorders
6. master gland of the body that regulates and coordinates the action of other endocrine glands and influences the growth and development of the body
7. hypersecretion of growth hormone after the epiphyses of bones have closed, resulting in normal stature of adults with enlarged hands, feet and facial features
8. condition caused by a deficiency or total absence of vasopressin secretion by the posterior pituitary

Fill in the Blank

1. increased appetite, muscle weakness, fatigue, palpitations, irritability, nervousness, sleep disorders, flushing, heat intolerance, tremors, altered menstrual flow, diarrhea, exopthalmus
2. Propylthiouracil (PTU), methimazole (Tapazole)
3. Beta-adrenergic blocking agents
4. Amiodarone
5. Graves' disease
6. calcium, phosphate
7. giantism, acromegaly
8. desmopressin acetate (DDAVP)

Multiple Choice

1. B	6. B
2. A	7. D
3. A	8. D
4. C	9. D
5. C	10. A

Multiple Response

1. A, B, E, F
2. A, D, E, F

Chapter 35

Definitions

1. complex disorder of carbohydrate, fat, and protein metabolism caused by lack or inefficient use of insulin in the body
2. formerly called insulin dependent diabetes mellitus, high blood sugar results from total lack of insulin
3. formerly called non-insuli-dependent diabetes mellitus, high blood sugar as a result of lack of insulin or the body's inability to utilize insulin efficiently
4. first injectable insulin that provides continuous dosing over a 24-hour period
5. also known as an insulin pump, provides a constant amount of insulin continuously throughout a 24-hour period by infusion of of insulin through a subcutaneous needle connected to the pump via tubing
6. class or oral antidiabetic medications that cause a decrease in blood sugar by stimulating insulin release in the pancreas, making it dependent on functioning beta cells
7. form of parenteral therapy for Type 2 diabetes mellitus
8. most common strength of insulin available; type of insulin and syringe used must match when administering the drug

Fill in the Blank

1. Diazoxide (Proglycem)
2. subcutaneous
3. NPH
4. 48
5. Acarbose (Precose)
6. 24
7. rosiglitazone (Avandia)
8. 6

Multiple Choice

1. C
2. A
3. C
4. C
5. A
6. B
7. D
8. A
9. C
10. B

Multiple Response

1. A, C, D, E
2. B, D, E, F

Chapter 36

Definitions

1. secreted by the testes in males and resulting in development of the external genitalia, deepening of the voice, and growth of hair in pubic, axillary, body, and facial areas
2. secreted by the ovaries of females and resulting in development of breast tissue, deposition of fat in the area of the thighs and hips, and hair growth in the pubic and axillary parts of the body
3. a completely synthetic estrogen that does not share the chemical structure of the natural estrogens,but exerts quite similar pharmacologic effects
4. consistent inability to obtain and maintain an erection sufficient for sexual intercourse

Fill in the Blank

1. anticoagulant, antidiabetic, anti-inflammatory corticosteroid

2. 7 days

3. thrombophlebitis

4. visual

5. cardiac arrest

Multiple Choice

1. C	6. C
2. B	7. C
3. A	8. A
4. B	9. D
5. C	10. B

Multiple Response

1. A, E, F

2. A, B

Chapter 37

Definitions

1. selective stimulants of uterine smooth muscle

2. an agent used to suppress lactation

3. agent used to stimulate uterine smooth muscle

4. agent used to inhibit the contractility of the uterine smooth muscle to prolong the gestational period

5. agent that stimulates beta$_2$ receptors in the uterus, thus relaxing the uterus

Fill in the Blank

1. 120, 160

2. Cervidil

3. methylergonovine maleate (Methergine)

4. drug-induced fever

5. left

Multiple Choice

1. A	6. D
2. D	7. D
3. B	8. D
4. A	9. A
5. D	10. C

Multiple Response

1. A, B, D, E

2. A, C, F

Chapter 38

Definitions
1. a medication containing weakened or dead antigens
2. administering an antigen, usually a vaccine, that has been diluted, weakened, or killed so it does not cause full disease symptoms
3. low molecular weight proteins that regulate the extent and duration of the immune and inflammatory response
4. drugs that suppress the immunological system of the body; primarily used to prevent organ rejection
5. one of the most effective immunosuppressant agents, responsible for many of the dramatic advances made in transplant surgery during the last two decades

Fill in the Blank
1. Immunology
2. Immunization
3. calcium gluconate, morphine sulfate
4. live attenuated
5. eggs, gelatin

Multiple Choice
1. A
2. D
3. D
4. D
5. B
6. A
7. D
8. D

Multiple Response
1. A, C, D, F
2. A, B, C

Chapter 39

Definitions
1. broad term encompassing many different related diseases all sharing the common characteristic of uncontrolled cell proliferation
2. drugs that exert their lethal effects by interfering with the cell cycle of both normal and malignant cells
3. agents that interfere with the chemical structure of DNA and cause abnormal chemical bonding between adjacent DNA molecules
4. drugs used in combination with chemotherapy, also known as rescue drugs, to combat specific adverse effects associated with particular antineoplastic agents
5. agents that bind to specific antigens on malignant lymphocytes resulting in lysis of cancer cells
6. agents that work by targeting and enhancing the immune system; they enhance the immunologic function of the host, destroy or interfere with the cellular activities of tumors, and promote the differentiation of stem cells
7. antineoplastic drugs that act by specifically interfering with cell division or miosis, the M phase of the cell cycle
8. agents that tend to concentrate in a specific tissue and emit damaging radiation, which destroys some or all of the tissue in which the drug is localized

Fill in the Blank
1. Epoetin
2. Pegfilgrastim
3. antiemmetics
4. palifermin
5. Xerostomia
6. G1, S, G2, M

Multiple Choice
1. C
2. A
3. C
4. C
5. B
6. D
7. A
8. B
9. C
10. A

Multiple Response
1. B, D, E
2. A, B, F

Chapter 40

Definitions
1. the iris occludes the anterior chamber structures of the eye and reduces outflow of aqueous humor
2. drugs that inhibit the action of carbonic anhydrase and are used in conjunction with topical agents to treat glaucoma
3. no change in chamber angle, but degenerative changes impeded the flow of aqueous humor
4. agents that rapidly reduce production of aqueous humor by withdrawing fluid from the body
5. medications used to stimulate adrenergic receptors in the eye
6. medications that cause constriction of the pupil
7. medications that prevent enzymatic destruction of acetylcholine within the eye by inhibiting cholinesterase, thereby resulting in miosis
8. medications that reduce the production of aqueous humor when applied topically
9. agent used for the treatment of fungal eye infections
10. dilation of the pupil

Fill in the Blank
1. dilate
2. constrict
3. cycloplegia
4. Natamycin
5. scarring of the retina and loss of vision
6. increased intraocular pressure
7. increased intraocular pressure
8. pilocarpine

Multiple Choice

1. A	6. B
2. B	7. B
3. A	8. C
4. C	9. C
5. A	10. A

Multiple Response

1. A, E, F
2. B, D

Chapter 41

Definitions

1. part of the ear where sound is conducted

2. part of the ear that contains the cohchlea and semicircular canals

3. a waxy substance that helps protect the ear canal

4. the outer, external component of the ear

5. the sensory organ of hearing

Fill in the Blank

1. otitis media

2. shorter, straighter

3. Wax emulsifiers

4. Antimicrobial

5. down, back

Multiple Choice

1. D	6. B
2. B	7. C
3. B	8. A
4. D	9. D
5. C	10. C

Multiple Response

1. A, B, C, D
2. A, B, E, F

Chapter 42

Definitions

1. medications that are oily substances that form an occlusive layer when applied to the skin to prevent further loss of moisture

2. agents that aid in removing excess keratin

3. agents that inhibit sensory nerve impulses and may contain antihistamines to decrease an immunological response

4. glands connected to hair follicles that are abundant on the head and face

5. layer of skin where new skin cells are formed

6. medications used to treat viral infections of the skin

7. glands connected to hair follicles that are not as widely dispersed as eccrine glands

8. premalignant skin disorders that commonly develop in fair-skinned individuals in the areas of the body that are heavily exposed to sunlight

Fill in the Blank

1. emollients

2. acne, warts, psoriasis, corns, calluses, fungal infections

3. pain, puritus

4. tinea

5. Candida albicans (Monilia)

Multiple Choice

1. A
2. B
3. D
4. C
5. A
6. C
7. B
8. C
9. B
10. D

Multiple Response

1. A, B, C, D
2. B, C, D